Production Development and Direction:

Chad Bennett, Dave Broome, Cindy Chang, Neysa Gordon, Mark Koops, Todd Nelson, Kim Niemi, J. D. Roth, Ben Silverman

NBCU, Reveille, 25/7 Productions, and 3Ball Productions would like to thank the many people who gave their time and energy to this project:

Jenna Alifante, Dave Altarescu, Stephen Andrade, Carole Angelo, Dana Arnett, Sebastian Attie, Nancy Bailey, *The Biggest Loser* contestants, Dave Bjerke, Maria Bohe, Jessa Bouso, Jen Busch, Joni Camacho, Jill Carmen, Scot Chastain, Hope Clarke, Ben Cohen, Jason Cooper, Steve Coulter, Dan Curran, Dr. Michael Dansinger, Camilla Dhanak, Jenny Ellis, Kat Elmore, John Farrell, Cheryl Forberg, Jeff Friedman, Jeff Gaspin, Christina Gaugler, Marc Graboff, Graham Greenlee, Bob Harper, Chris Harris, Robyn Hennessey, Shelli Hill, Dr. Robert Huizenga, Jill Jarosz, Helen Jorda, Adam Kaloustian, Alex Katz, Allison Kaz, Loretta Kraft, Chris Krogermeier, Laura Kuhn, Beth Lamb, Todd Lubin, Roni Lubliner, Alan Lundgren, Carole MacDonal, Rebecca Marks, Joaquin Mesa, Jillian Michaels, Gregg Michaelson, John Miller, Ann Morteo, Kam Naderi, Gabriela Navarro, Julie Nugent, Trae Patton, Jerry Petry, Ellie Prezant, Ed Prince, Lee Rierson, Karen Rinaldi, Melissa Roberson, Beth Roberts, Maria Rodale, Jessica Roth, Joe Schlosser, Leslie Schwartz, Robin Shallow, Carrie Simons, Mitch Steele, Lee Straus, Kelia Tardiff, Paul Teledgy, Deborah Thomas, Julie True, Liza Whitcraft, Julie Will, Yong Yam, Jeff Zucker

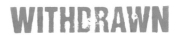

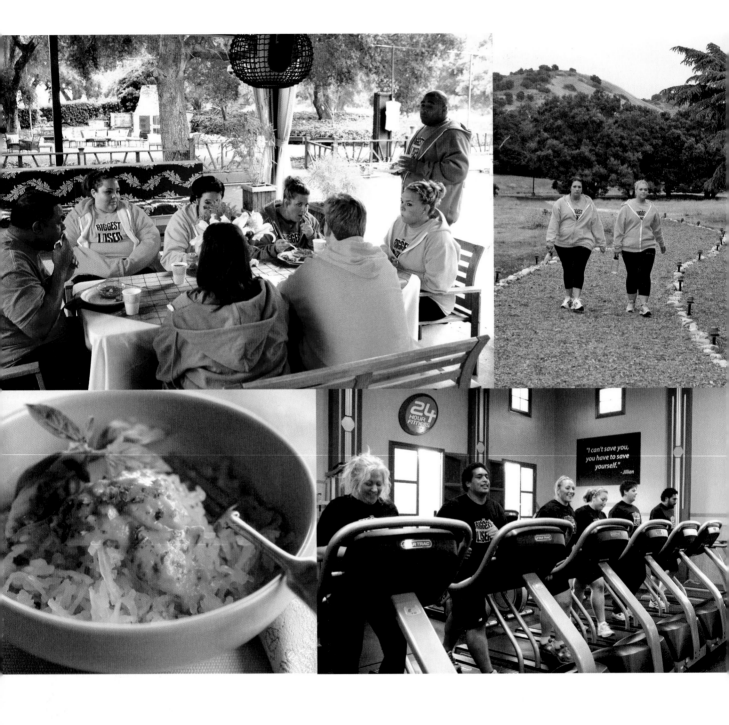

Contents

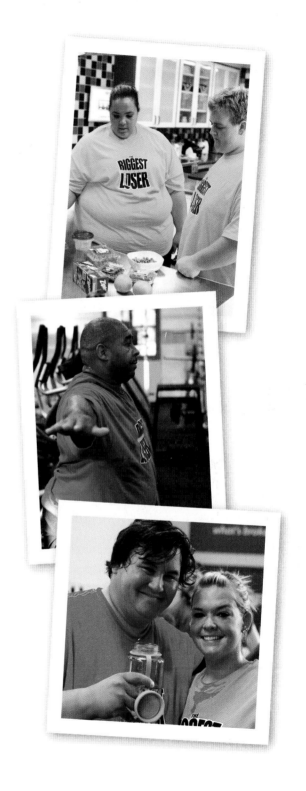

Introduction

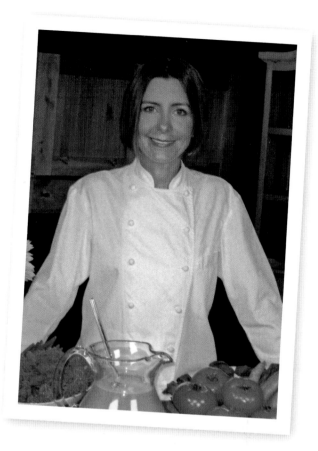

When I opened my newspaper on a recent morning, I read something that shocked me: Over the past year, our obesity rates did not decrease *in any state* in America. It's hard for me to believe, because as the nutritionist for *The Biggest Loser,* I see and hear so many weight-loss success stories every day—and not just from contestants, but from viewers as well.

I first meet the contestants at the start of each new season of the show, when they sit down with me for a comprehensive nutrition consultation. During these meetings, I have the opportunity to learn about each individual's unique history and struggles, including their typical eating habits and their past attempts to lose weight. What's interesting is that no matter how different each person's story is, almost all of them share many of the same issues. By now, I can almost predict some of the answers I'll receive to the questions I ask.

After eight wonderful seasons with the show, I've learned a lot about the common difficulties and obstacles many Americans face when it comes to their eating habits and attempts at weight management. Among these issues, I've identified 10 key factors that I believe play a vital role in weight gain and poor overall health. I've found that most of our contestants:

1. Had absolutely no idea how many calories their bodies really needed (or how many they consumed each day).

2. Frequently skipped breakfast and other meals.

3. Didn't eat enough fruits or vegetables.

4. Didn't eat enough lean protein.

5. Didn't eat enough whole grains.

6. Ate too much "white stuff," such as white flour, white pasta, white sugar, white rice, and simple carbohydrates.

7. Didn't plan their meals in advance and often found themselves grabbing something on the go, which they ate standing up, in the car, or at their desks.

8. Drank too many of their calories (some people consumed their daily calorie budgets in sugary drinks alone!) but didn't drink enough water or milk.

9. Didn't get enough exercise (if any).

10. Prioritized other things—such as their families, friends, and jobs—over their own health and well-being.

If you're trying to lose weight, you're probably all too familiar with many of these challenges. This book provides the tools you need to get started on your own transformation. A lot of people are afraid that creating a healthier lifestyle will be too hard or too expensive or that it will require too much time and effort. The idea behind Simple Swaps is to make getting healthy a less daunting challenge. Living a healthier life doesn't mean you have to change everything at once—it begins with small, manageable steps. A good place to start is to swap some of your daily habits and choices for healthier versions. For example, you might swap your daily glass of fruit juice for a piece of whole fruit, or swap your sweet afternoon treat from the coffee shop for a satisfying snack that combines protein and carbohydrates to give you a boost of energy.

I created 100 Simple Swaps and more than 30 mouthwatering recipes for this book based on my experience and success with *The Biggest Loser* contestants and the common struggles most people face when it comes to weight loss. Many of these recommendations are the same ones I give the contestants when they come to see me on that first day at *The Biggest Loser* ranch. Throughout the book, you'll find not only my recommendations and advice, but tips from the contestants themselves, who know firsthand how tough it can be to fit lifestyle changes into a busy schedule, and who have incorporated these swaps into their weight-loss efforts.

Whether you're looking to shed just a few pounds, lose a significant amount of weight, or simply maintain a healthy weight, these Simple Swaps will not only help you keep fit, but also ensure that you're getting the nutrients you need for optimal health and wellness. Swapping one unhealthy food, habit, or lifestyle choice for another, better one is where it all begins.

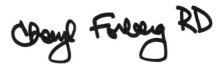

Notes to the Chef from the Chef

In my seven seasons with the show, I quickly learned that our contestants, like most other Americans, are *very* busy people. With that in mind, most of the Simple Swap recipes are fairly easy to prepare. There aren't too many fancy ingredients or expensive kitchen tools to buy. However, portion size is always key to staying within your calorie budget, so measuring tools are a must. They include liquid measuring cups, dry measuring cups, measuring spoons, and a food scale (see Chapter 2 for more details).

Here are a few of my other must-have kitchen tools.

Tools

Squeeze bottles I love to keep a variety of squeeze bottles on hand in the kitchen. Not only do they allow you to aim, shoot, and squeeze small amounts of sauces or dressings into a pretty design on your plate (instead of pouring out a big glob), but the narrower the opening, the slower the pour, meaning that you use less dressing or sauce. And a smaller amount translates into fewer calories. I even like to put purchased bottled dressings and sauces into squeeze bottles, because they deliver a much smaller portion and they're so easy to use.

Spray bottles Cooking oil spray is used throughout this book to minimize use of added fat. Rather than using aerosolized cans, I recommend purchasing an oil spray bottle, which you can find in most health food stores. Fill it with your own fresh oils as needed. For regular baking and sautéing, fill the spray bottle with a mild-flavored oil. Cooking oils can be stored in a cool, dark place for up to 4 months. Because they are composed of highly unsaturated fats, they will turn rancid within several months after opening. Buying a large bottle with a great price tag is not the best option, since you'll be adding less oil to your cooking. When in doubt of your oil's freshness, throw it out and open a fresh bottle. One tablespoon of rancid oil can ruin the flavor of an entire recipe.

Handheld zester/grater This multitasking tool gets regular workouts in my kitchen. Did you know that more than 50 percent of the vitamin C in citrus fruits is in the peel? For that reason, I like to grate the zest of a lemon or orange or whichever citrus fruit I'm using (or eating) into a pitcher of water, or onto my salad or cereal. I love the citrus flavor, and I know I'm getting an extra bang of vitamin C and not wasting any part of the fruit. The other use for this tool is grating hard cheeses, such as Parmesan or Romano. Losing weight does not mean saying good-bye to cheese. Yes, it's high in calories, but a little bit goes a long way, and this tool allows you to grate a fine dusting of cheese on your salad or whole grain pasta without breaking your calorie budget.

Ingredients

In terms of grocery shopping, it's a no-brainer to say that organic is better, but I know not everyone can afford that option. If you can, great. If not, just be sure to shop for produce that looks fresh and, when possible, is in season. One thing you'll learn as you become more comfortable in the kitchen is that the quality of the food you prepare is a function of the quality of its ingredients. Buy the freshest and best-quality ingredients you can afford.

If you've been a hard-core fast-food and processed-food eater, switching over to *The Biggest Loser* eating plan (and doing all the exercise!) will really make a difference in how you taste and appreciate food. When you swap out salty, sugary, fried, and processed foods for clean foods made from fresh ingredients, your palate will notice the difference. You'll spend more time reading food labels and assessing produce at the grocery store than you ever did looking at a drive-thru menu!

I'm always adding to my repertoire of ingredients, always looking for new products for my pantry, and I've included most of my current favorites in the Simple Swap recipes.

Other ingredient and shopping tips:

- Buying seasonal and local produce will help ensure better value as well as better flavor.
- Fresh fruits and vegetables are optimal, but frozen are also perfectly fine.
- Buy less, waste less. If you're buying more fresh produce than you used to (and you probably will be), you may find it beneficial to tack on an extra trip to the market each week to be sure that you use up your purchases instead of stocking up and allowing some of them to go to waste. This is particularly true when you're getting started and aren't quite sure how long all those fresh veggies will last.
- If your store doesn't carry everything you need (such as fat-free Greek-style yogurt, fat-free ricotta cheese, and turkey breast), be sure to ask your grocer to order it. These days all stores want to retain their loyal customers, and if you're looking for a particular ingredient, chances are that other customers are, too—just ask!
- Shop with a list and stick to it! It curbs impulsive purchases and cuts down grocery bills.
- If you're following a sodium-restricted diet, you can eliminate the small amounts of salt in the Simple Swap recipes. (Conversely, if you don't have any restrictions, you can feel free to enhance the seasonings to your taste.)
- When possible, try to use fresh herbs instead of dried—the flavor is much more robust. That said, dried herbs do last longer. If dried herbs are your only option, remember that 1 teaspoon of dried herbs equals approximately 1 tablespoon of fresh herbs.
- You'll note that several of the recipes in this book include pure vanilla extract, one of my all-time favorite ingredients! Though a good-quality product may seem expensive, a little bit goes a long way. I always have a small dropper bottle (from the health food store) on hand, filled with vanilla extract. I use it to add a few drops to my lattes or to make my own unsweetened vanilla yogurt at home.

Cooking Methods

I have a lot to say about the importance of good fats in a healthy diet in Chapter 7. Because fat is so rich in calories, it's important to make your choices carefully. I like to eat my good fats in the form of avocados, nuts, seeds, and a little olive oil here and there. In terms of cooking, I can really keep the calorie count down when I focus on methods that do not require added fat.

Dry-heat cooking uses hot air or fat for heat transference. The cooking methods used in this book require minimal or no added fat. Using nonstick cookware and ensuring that the stove or oven is set to the right temperature are essential to successful dry-heat cooking.

Dry-Heat Methods

- **Baking** This method cooks food in an oven at a controlled temperature, usually in the range of 200° to 500°F, which is considerably lower than broiling and grilling temperatures. For this reason, baking usually takes longer. Also, since the hot air circulating around the pan is what actually cooks the food, don't crowd the oven without expecting the baking time to increase. Opt for nonstick bakeware so there's no need to grease the pan or add extra oil.

- **Roasting** Like baking, roasting takes place inside an oven, where food is surrounded by heat in a closed environment. The resulting coloring, from light to deep golden brown, adds depth to the food's flavor and richness to the color of any pan juices.

- **Broiling** This method involves placing food directly under a heat source, such as an open flame or an electric heating element. Cooking is usually accomplished rapidly, since the temperature is quite hot. In addition, the food's surface will brown and can easily char. Your undivided attention is required here, because this method is quick!

- **Grilling** This style of cooking places food directly *over* a flame, which can be maintained by charcoal, gas, or different types of wood. The temperature range frequently used is 400° to 500°F, which allows the food to cook very quickly, depending on how close it is to the heat. Like broiling, this method results in browning and a crispy exterior, and, depending on the heat source, can enhance your food with smoky flavor.

- **Dry sautéing** To sauté a food is to fry it, typically in a moderate amount of oil, butter, or both. *Sauté* means "to jump" in French. This method is very quick and therefore involves high heat. Using a good nonstick pan and an optional mist of oil, we can accomplish the same result with just a trace of fat. The key is to ensure that the pan is hot before adding the food, to reduce the chances of sticking. A good nonstick skillet is required, and an oil mister makes "oil rationing" a breeze!

Wet-heat cooking uses hot liquid (typically water, broth, butter, or oil) to cook a food. The food may be fully submerged in liquid, suspended over it, or submerged in only a shallow portion of liquid. When water is used as the liquid, no added fat is needed to cook the food.

Wet-Heat Methods

- **Poaching** This method involves placing food directly into water or another liquid, which may be seasoned. The item to be poached, such as a salmon fillet, an egg, or a chicken breast, is submerged in hot liquid and simmered just until cooked. Although there are special pieces of equipment available for poaching fish and eggs, a shallow saucepan works very well. Try the Garlicky Poached Chicken Breasts with Ginger and Onion on page 93.

- **Pressure cooking** This method requires the use of a special piece of equipment called a pressure cooker, which is a heavy pot with a very tight-fitting lid. This pressure chamber allows food to cook quickly, and drastically reduces cooking time. No added fat is required for pressure cooking.
- **Steaming** In this technique, food is placed in a metal or bamboo basket over boiling water, which allows steam to circulate around the food and cook it through. You can also use *The Biggest Loser* steamer, the same tool used by contestants at the ranch. Although water works well as a steaming liquid, you may use fat-free broths as well. Herbs and spices, such as garlic or ginger, enhance flavor when added to boiling liquid.

Enhancements

Because fat has a distinctive mouth feel and carries flavor, cutting back on it can quickly change the texture and appeal of your favorite dishes. It's key to understand the value of enhancements in healthy cooking. Enhancements include the addition of an ingredient either to . . .

- compensate for the loss or reduction of another
- achieve optimal nutritional balance (by adding fiber or protein, for example), or
- most important, add flavor or texture!

This is perhaps the most essential and least understood aspect of healthy cooking. One of the most valuable uses of enhancements in lower-fat cooking is to add flavor and texture, both of which are lost when we reduce or eliminate fat. Let's face it, it's not easy to stick to a new way of eating if it doesn't taste good. Perhaps the best example of enhancement is the addition of herbs and spices, which really gives us unlimited creativity. The addition of enhancements may take place during different stages of the cooking process.

In the initial stages, enhancements may be made with a marinade or a dry rub. A marinade is a liquid often containing an oil, an acid (such as lemon juice, wine, or vinegar), and a variety of herbs or spices. The acidic component usually helps to tenderize the meat, though care must be taken not to use too much acid, because it will break down the proteins and change the texture. Salt should not be used in a marinade, because it draws the moisture out of the meat. The purpose of a marinade, then, is not only to tenderize, but also to add flavor, or enhance it! A dry rub is a mixture of herbs, spices, and sometimes a paste of onions and garlic. Because they don't contain liquids, dry rubs do not tenderize, but they are fat free and are great flavor boosters!

Spices or herbs may also be incorporated *during* the cooking process. And fresh herbs may be sprinkled over a dish as a garnish or at the last moment to retain their fresh flavors. The possibilities of using enhancements are numerous. But when we consider seasonings borrowed from regional and ethnic cuisines, the options are endless.

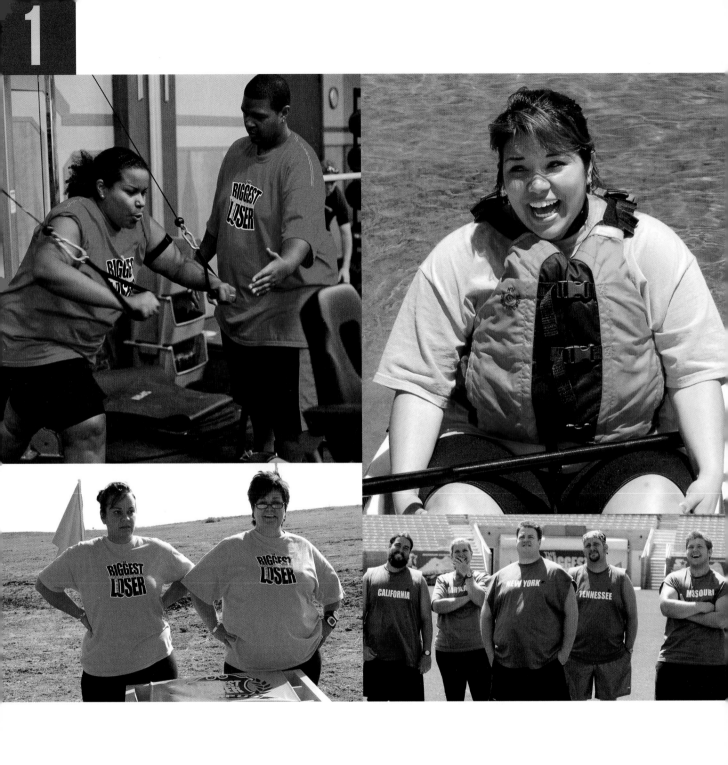

Swapping the Ranch for Life at Home

The *Biggest Loser* campus is not a luxury resort, and getting healthy is no vacation—it requires hard work, focus, and discipline. But on the ranch, contestants are allowed the freedom to focus exclusively on their health and weight-loss goals, without all the other responsibilities of "real life"—jobs, kids, homes to maintain, obligations to fulfill. In the context of fierce competition, drive and focus are easy to summon. And what better motivation to maintain that sense of discipline than to be weighed each week (in spandex!) in front of a television audience of millions?

But eventually, the cameras shut off, the lights dim, and the contestants go back home to a life that doesn't include access to superstar trainers, a campus bordered by mountains and hiking trails, and a beautiful kitchen that's always stocked with healthy foods. What happens then? How do former *Biggest Loser* contestants maintain their weight loss—and their focus—in the real world?

In the pages that follow, you'll have the opportunity to catch up with some of your favorite *Biggest Losers* from across the seasons and learn how they've dealt with the challenges that life's thrown their way since they returned home from the ranch. While they've all encountered obstacles to their weight maintenance and fitness regimens, they've also devised strategies to help them overcome those obstacles and honor the dedication they made at the ranch to a lifetime of health. For each of them, it's the everyday choices—the small decisions—that really count. Changing unhealthy habits, opting for healthier choices, and making Simple Swaps are essential to their success—and to yours.

The Guy with the Big Hair

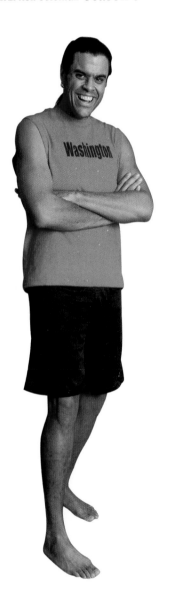

Starting weight: 358 pounds

Height: 6'4"

Home: Gresham, Oregon

Finale weight: 197 pounds

Weight today: 235 pounds

You may remember Season 3's Ken Coleman as the tall guy with the big hair—and the big, deep, booming voice. Ken says the only thing he can remember about his first few days on the ranch is thinking, "How am I going to get out of this?" For 15 years he had been making excuses not to exercise—but *The Biggest Loser* trainers weren't buying those excuses.

Ken quickly realized he wasn't going to get out of anything, so he might as well give it his all. So he started moving and stopped complaining. And not only did he get himself going, but he also encouraged his wife, Amy, to start making better choices. By the time he arrived home from the ranch, she had lost 40 pounds, and she's since lost an additional 35 pounds!

Shortly after Ken returned home from Season 3, he was rushed to the hospital for an emergency appendectomy. Doctors told him his weight loss had made the operation much more successful than it would have been otherwise. "Losing the weight probably saved my life," says Ken.

Today he works as a personal trainer, helping his clients find their own paths back to health. "The biggest hurdle I run into with coaching clients is that they don't feel ready yet. Well, they are ready. They wouldn't be coming to me if they weren't. I tell them you just have to quit using excuses as a crutch. Just get out there and get moving and the mind will follow."

He also counsels his clients to understand that these changes are for life. "You can't get your weight where you want it, then go back to old ways of eating. Once you get your momentum going, don't stop. If you stop, you risk finding yourself at square one again."

Ken says one of the most valuable qualities he brings to others battling their excess weight is that he's been there. And he's willing to listen. "I don't know everything about weight loss there is to know; it's an ongoing educational process. But I always sit down and take the time to listen, finding ways for them to start making minor changes slowly and setting achievable goals."

The first thing Coleman asks his clients to do is to write down everything they eat, not recording calories but simply getting their intake down on paper. "Then we can take a look at it and start making adjustments.

"Acknowledging that you want help," says Ken, "and being open to what you'll hear are keys to turning your life around."

Ken's Simple Swaps

■ Swap food that comes in a box for fresh food that doesn't need packaging. "Stay away from processed foods," says Ken. "Buy fresh and cook it all up at once, storing some in bags in the freezer for later. Make your own meals."

■ Swap skipping meals for eating throughout the day. "It may sound odd to say that to an overweight person, but you have to eat meals and snacks each day. Just don't overindulge at any of them."

■ Swap big goals for small ones. "Who's going to give up their job and work out 10 hours a day?" asks Ken. "Set goals you can achieve," he advises.

■ Swap ignorance for bliss. "Learn how to read nutrition labels and understand what proteins do, what carbs do," says Ken. Understanding nutrition will help you make better food choices moving forward.

A 9-Month Detour

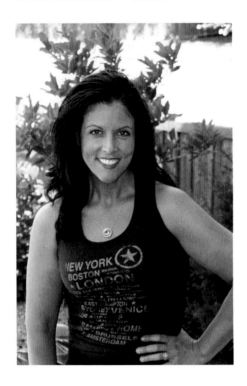

Starting weight: 245 pounds

Height: 5'4"

Home: Shakopee, Minnesota

Finale weight: 145 pounds

Weight today: 162 pounds (postpregnancy)

Goal weight: 145 pounds

Jennifer Eisenbarth proved early on that you could be a *Biggest Loser* off the ranch. Six days into Season 3, she was eliminated. "I wasn't sure how I was going to do it on my own, but I knew I had committed to it," she says. "I had spent months telling the producers of the show that I was ready to lose the weight. So I knew I was committed. I went home and kept eating clean, exercising, and being consistent." And it worked. She returned to her season's finale 100 pounds lighter.

She didn't find postfinale maintenance that difficult at first. For a few months, she kept her weight consistent by doing three or four workouts a week and even added about 400 more calories to her daily diet to maintain a healthy weight. Then one day she noticed her waist was inexplicably a few inches bigger. As it turned out, another little Eisenbarth was on the way. Jennifer was thrilled at the thought of expanding her family—but not at the thought of her body expanding. "I am part of the third generation of an obese family. I had worked so hard to finally lose the weight, and I felt extremely anxious about the impending weight gain."

So what did she do? "I put away the scale. For the health of my child, I didn't want to know the number. I'd go to the doctor's and step on the scale backward." What she did know was that she could lose it again. But she needed to keep from stressing about the fact that her body was growing and gaining, as it was supposed to.

She says that for her entire pregnancy, she never looked at the scale once. In fact, it was only recently that she learned the actual number of pounds she gained: 91. Her son, Tate, was born healthy but colicky, so the next 8 or 9 months were devoted to tending to him and her two older daughters. Finally, in November 2008, her husband asked her what she wanted for her birthday, and her answer was "Dr. Huizenga." She enrolled in a support group of patients guided by Dr. Rob Huizenga, a medical expert for *The Biggest Loser,* and today she is within 17 pounds of her goal weight of 145.

These days Jen wakes up at 5:00 each morning so that she can get in a workout before her husband leaves for work at 8:00 a.m. "Sometimes I'm exhausted and want to hit snooze, but the reality is that I always feel better after working out. And there's something very spiritual about working out early in the morning. It centers me for the day." And if there's a family walk at the end of the day, "that's gravy," she says.

She is careful, especially as the mother of two young girls, never to use the word *diet.* "I call it 'training down.' Mommy's 'training down.' My 5-year-old and I were out walking the other day, and she ran ahead to the light post. She turned around and said, 'I'm getting strong, just like Mommy.' My husband turned to me and said, 'You are giving her that gift.'"

Jen's Simple Swaps

- Swap someone else's voice for your own. "We're told what's acceptable and what's not by others. But listen to *your* voice. Figure out what works for you."
- Swap unplanned evening time for rules. "After I get the kids to bed, I don't let myself wander into the kitchen. It's off-limits. Otherwise the temptation is, 'It's quiet; let's go have something to eat as a reward.' If I want a glass of water, my husband can go get it for me!"
- Swap "I can't have this" for "I *can* have this." "Make a list of all the things you *can* eat. List all the veggies and fruit and lean protein and dairy. There's a lot you can have and be satisfied."
- Swap withholding for providing. "I don't forbid sweets for my kids. But I don't buy unhealthy snacks, either. If I don't buy it and it's not around the house, they don't eat it."
- Swap a kid-free kitchen zone for cooking helpers. "We eat shrimp boats that I let the kids make themselves. Take cooked shrimp and put them in a long leaf of romaine lettuce. Top with mango salsa, a little shredded cheese, and a squeeze of lime. The kids love it."
- Swap self-criticism for self-love. "What we say to ourselves really affects our whole being. Things we would never say to other people we often say to ourselves. Why would we do that? People need to talk to themselves with love and respect."

Amy and Marty Wolff

UPDATE: Amy Hildreth Wolff and Marty Wolff Season 3

Amy

Starting weight: 260 pounds

Height: 5'10"

Home: Omaha, Nebraska

Finale weight: 154 pounds

Weight today: "That's between me and my scale."

Marty

Starting weight: 365 pounds

Height: 6'0"

Home: Omaha, Nebraska

Finale weight: 219 pounds

Weight today: 255 pounds

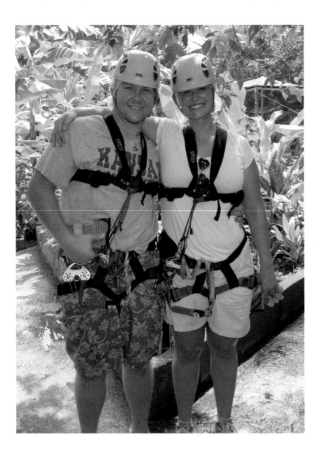

While contestants don't necessarily come to the ranch looking for love, *The Biggest Loser* has produced more marriages than most dating reality TV shows! One of those happy couples is Amy Hildreth and Marty Wolff, who met during Season 3 and began dating soon afterward. Today they are also the proud parents of Blaine Patrick Wolff, a "firecracker baby," as his mom calls him, born July 4, 2009.

Marty and Amy have moved their family back to their hometown of Omaha, Nebraska (after they started dating, they found out that they had been born 10 miles apart), and created a corporate wellness program called Reality Wellness. "We have a boot camp we run in Omaha," says Amy, "and we focus on all sizes and shapes. We work with people who have 200 pounds to lose to people who have run marathons.

"Our message is that even though we were on a show and it was about a number, it's really about learning healthy habits," says Amy. "Goals change," says Marty, who's comfortable with the fact that he gained some weight after his season's finale. "My weight at the finale was the result of someone who worked out 4 to 8 hours a day. But it's a big healthy step when you adjust to real life and realize the weight at which you feel healthy."

Amy, too, is no longer fond of using a number to define her health. "I don't really like to put numbers out there," she says. "The important thing is I've found a weight where I feel healthy and happy and that's sustainable. That's what counts. I didn't want to live a life of working out 6 hours a day to stay at my finale weight."

What also counts is their new bundle of joy, whom they're looking forward to introducing to their active lifestyle. "We are going to be very well equipped now as role models," says his mom. "We can't wait to take him hiking and kayaking, to have fun outdoors."

Today Amy is focused on losing her baby weight after her C-section forced her to take it easy for 8 to 10 weeks. "I gained a lot more pregnancy weight than I planned," she says, "but my doctor told me I was going to be fine. He knows I know how to take it off. I have that confidence now." Now she's back to working out 6 days a week for a couple of hours a day and keeping a food journal. "We eat tons of veggies and fruit. Marty's a great cook, so he usually cooks for both of us."

The Wolffs are looking forward to enjoying their new family and continuing to help others find fit and healthy lives.

Amy and Marty's Simple Swaps

- Swap focusing on limitations for focusing on potential. "People are looking for an opportunity to be involved in something greater than themselves," says Marty. Getting healthy leads to a fuller participation in life.
- Swap wanting for needing. "When we think about dinner," says Amy, "we don't necessarily think about what we want to have, but what our bodies need. That takes away the emotions behind the eating and focuses more on nurturing your body."
- Swap looking for a finish line to committing to a new lifestyle. "[Trainer] Bob Harper used to say if you're here to lose 10 to 20 pounds, you're here for the wrong reason," says Marty. "Weight loss is a long-term commitment."
- Swap eating to endure upsets for movement. "If you're feeling upset over something," says Amy, "go take a walk or ride a bike to jolt yourself out of your negative thinking. Getting out of the house can help you get back on track."
- Swap inertia for finding new ways to move. "We look at every errand as a way to burn calories," says Amy. "Instead of trying to unload all the groceries at once, we willingly run back and forth, unloading a few at a time."

A Million Times Happier

Starting weight: 279 pounds

Height: 5'6"

Home: Philadelphia

Finale weight: 174 pounds

Weight today: 180 pounds

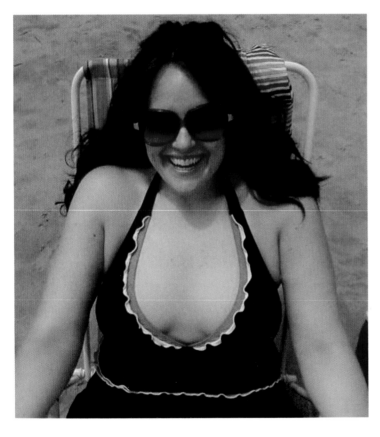

Everyone has to answer the "why" of their overeating, says Nicole Michalik, before they can do something about it. "For me," she says, "it was about entitlement. If my skinny friends could eat at Wendy's, why couldn't I?" Turns out that one reason was her hypothyroidism, or underactive thyroid, which keeps her metabolism in a slower state than normal. Dr. Rob Huizenga, a medical expert for *The Biggest Loser*, gave her a reality check. "He basically said, 'You're going to have to work harder.' I finally started to accept the reality of my situation, that I would have to work harder and really watch what I ate. These are the cards I was dealt."

Nicole has turned those cards into a winning hand by keeping the weight off through a steady and consistent schedule of workouts (an hour and a half, 6 days a week!) and keeping a very close eye on what she eats. "It's just a part of my life, like brushing my teeth. You wouldn't wake up in the morning and say, 'Oh, I don't feel like brushing my teeth this morning,' would you?"

Now if her friends go to Wendy's, she goes to the salad bar next door. "There's always a grocery store with a salad bar somewhere nearby, no matter where your friends want to eat. Load up on veggies and garbanzo beans. You can find a way around the situation."

Another strategy Nicole uses when she wants a higher-calorie food is to eat the simplest version possible. "If you're at a pizza place, get a salad and one slice of pizza if you really want that. But make it just a plain slice—don't get it loaded up with stuff."

Today, she says she's the happiest she's ever been in her life, as well as the healthiest. "I'm not afraid anymore. I don't have to tell people that I can't go to an amusement park because I won't fit in the rides or I can't go zip-lining because I won't fit in the harness. I'm sitting on planes now with my legs crossed—and that never gets old! After years of being fat, of feeling crazy, miserable, and insecure, I finally feel like myself."

In addition to her job as a disc jockey in Philadelphia, she's enjoying speaking to groups about health, especially kids. "How do you teach a 12-year-old if he's out with friends who want to eat junk? He has to say no. It's like smoking or drinking; it's not good for you. If your friends don't like you for holding back from harmful behaviors, then they're not your friends. This is about making you feel better about yourself."

"As Bob [Harper] would say, knowledge is power," says Nicole. "Once you're educated, the possibilities are endless."

Nicole's Simple Swaps

- Swap caramel-, nougat-, and nut-laden candy bars for a couple of pieces of good, plain chocolate. "Simpler is better," says Nicole.
- Swap hating exercise for loving it. "Find what works for you. For me, a group setting is best. And I love having music in the background."
- Swap always eating the birthday cake for *occasionally* eating the birthday cake. "There's always going to be someone having a birthday. You don't have to eat a slice of cake every single time."
- Swap narrow thinking for broadening your palate. "I come from a meat-and-potatoes upbringing, but I've learned to love all kinds of new healthy foods, like sushi!"

"He Loves Me Fat and Loves Me Skinny"

UPDATE: Bette-Sue Burklund **Season 5**

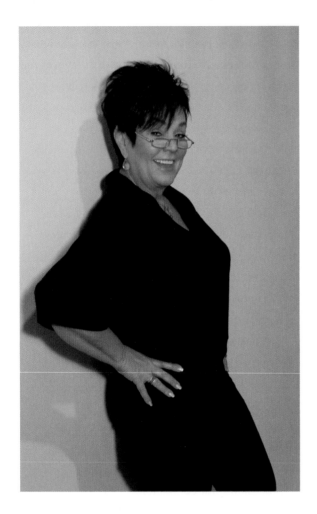

Starting weight: 261 pounds

Height: 5'5"

Home: Mesa, Arizona

Finale weight: 186 pounds

Weight today: 167 pounds

Bette-Sue Burklund, mother and teammate of Season 5's grand prize winner and superathlete Ali Vincent, admits that she hates to exercise. When she went on the show with her daughter, she swears she "didn't know how much hell it would be." But it looks as if hell has led to heaven.

Today, Bette-Sue is well below her finale weight and has kept it off, despite her aversion to the gym. "Most things I enjoy are sedentary," she says. "I love to quilt. I love to do needlepoint and play on my computer." But she says she gets a lot of exercise from just from running up and down the stairs in her home ("because I can't remember where anything is anymore") and playing with her grandkids.

Bette-Sue keeps a laserlike focus on what she eats. At 54, she says, she can't afford to get sloppy about her calorie intake. "I don't deny myself things I like; I just eat little portions. If I want a few potato chips, I count them out." And if she's going to eat a potato chip, she wants a *real* potato chip. "If I'm going to cheat, I'm going to cheat good," she laughs. "I know the number of calories I'm taking in."

But there are some foods she tries to stay away from, including pasta. "Eating has a lot to do with maturity and immediate gratification," she says. "I like to shop and buy what I want when I want it. And that used to be my relationship with food. But now I eat more slowly and in smaller quantities."

Although age may bring a slower metabolism and afflictions such as arthritis, she sees her age as an advantage overall. "I've been through the heavy-duty life stuff. I don't worry about where I fit in in this world. And I've been patient. It took me longer to lose the weight, but I can handle that."

Since losing the weight, she's been able to enjoy a more active lifestyle. She's looking forward to going on church missions with her husband after they retire, knowing that she now has the stamina and energy to undertake such trips. And she gets a kick out of her husband's admiration. "I was walking in front of him in a store the other day, and he said, 'You really are thin.' Then I had to shake it a little!"

Life as the mother of the show's first female *Biggest Loser* was a little surreal at first. "I was in awe of Ali, but it was hard living in her shadow. People didn't notice my weight loss compared to hers." But Bette-Sue has persevered and appreciates the panorama of her life. "I'm not unconscious in my life. I'm happy. I have fabulous children and grandchildren. I love my husband; we are so lucky we found each other. He loves me fat and loves me skinny. I have my faith. My mom. It's all good."

Bette-Sue's Simple Swaps

- Swap eating in bed for doing needlepoint in bed. Now, instead of eating late at night when she's bored or restless, Bette-Sue keeps her hands busy and her mind occupied with needlepoint.
- Swap skipping breakfast for eating breakfast. "I always eat first thing in the morning. I used to go all day and not eat until 3 or 4 in the afternoon, and then I would keep eating until I went to bed."
- Swap eating your whole meal for packing some of it up first. "I'll cook up a meal and immediately pack most of it up and put it in the fridge. My husband says it's packed up before he can sit down and eat it!"
- Swap defeat for confidence. "Believe in yourself to become what you want and to have what you deserve in your life."

Shedding Baby Weight at Boot Camp

UPDATE: Neill and Amanda Harmer Season 5

Amanda

Starting weight: 204 pounds

Height: 5'2"

Home: Bethany, Oklahoma

Finale weight: 140 pounds

Weight today: 150 pounds (postpregnancy)

Goal weight: 135 pounds

Neill Harmer

Starting weight: 317 pounds

Height: 5'10"

Home: Bethany, Oklahoma

Finale weight: 229 pounds

Weight today: 220 pounds

Maintained weight loss: 1.5 years

Two months after the Season 5 live finale, Amanda Harmer received news that would change her approach to weight maintenance—and her life in general: She was pregnant! "I was a little scared," she laughs. After returning home from the finale, she had dropped another 5 pounds, achieving her goal weight of 135 pounds. But baby daughter Eily, born in January 2009, wasn't going to let her maintain that weight for long.

"I gained 60 pounds during my pregnancy. Not what I planned," Amanda says. Her recovery was complicated by some medical problems, and she was not allowed to exercise for 15 weeks after Eily's birth. As a result, Amanda was extra careful with her eating. "Even though I couldn't work out, I lost a lot of weight by eating clean, journaling, and counting calories. I watched my sugar and soda intake," she says.

Once she could exercise again, Amanda got herself right back on track by teaching boot camp classes at night. "That's my time. Neill comes home and watches the kids, and I head off to the gym. I get my workout in, *and* I get paid!" she says.

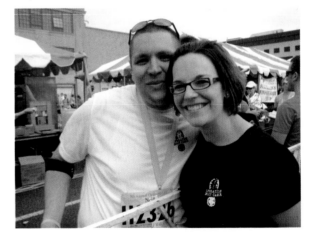

Neill is also maintaining an active lifestyle post-*Biggest Loser*. He's become an endurance athlete and has made fitness a focal point of his life. "I have at least one triathlon, mostly sprint ones, planned each month until the end of the year, when I'll have an Olympic-distance triathlon," Neill says. "My goal next year is a full marathon and a half Ironman triathlon," he adds. And Neill says it's the training he really loves. "I get up at 5:15 most mornings for a run or bike ride. Plus I lift weights. Once you get to a certain point, if you don't work out, you don't feel good."

For Neill, completing the triathlons is a matter of heart as well as body. A few years before he was cast for the show, the idea of competing in a triathlon so intrigued him that he bought a new pair of shoes to train for it. But nothing happened. He just couldn't get his training off the ground.

"Every time I finish a triathlon now," he says, "I get emotional. When I finished my first 5-K run, I could barely contain myself. I couldn't believe I had just done it. I remembered the years and years of thinking about triathlons and not being able to do them."

The healthy Harmers are passing their love of physical activity onto their children, as well. Neill says that they've even made their family vacations more active. "In the past, we would have just gone somewhere and sat around, eating. This year we're going canoeing in Arkansas."

Neill and Amanda's Simple Swaps

■ Swap your car for a bike. "I ride my bike to work, about 4 miles, but sometimes I take the long way home. I might go around the lake near our house and make the trip home 20 miles," says Neill

■ Swap excuses for intention. Neil says, "We've been to *The Biggest Loser* casting calls, and people ask us how to lose weight. You just have to make yourself do it. No one is going to do it for you."

■ Swap potato chips for fruit. "We don't keep stuff like chips around the house," says Amanda. "The kids don't even have the opportunity to ask for it."

■ Swap fast food once a week for once a month. Kids are kids, after all, and Amanda says, "We're not going to forbid our kids to eat fast food. But we limit our visits to once a month."

■ Swap ambiguity for goals. Despite all of his competitive training, Neill says, "I know I'll never be an elite athlete. But each triathlon I compete in, I give myself a time goal." Setting goals motivates you to perform your hardest.

Believe It, Be It

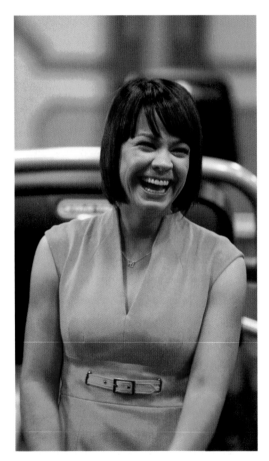

Starting weight: 234 pounds

Height: 5'5"

Home: Phoenix, Arizona

Finale weight: 122 pounds

Weight today: 125 pounds

When it comes to maintaining a healthy, active lifestyle, it's hard to think of a more motivated or enthusiastic person than Ali Vincent. The energy and determination she used to win the title of the first female *Biggest Loser* has not diminished one bit since Season 5's live finale, in which she proved pink was the color of victory.

These days, in addition to training for various races and keeping herself at peak performance, Ali also speaks to groups of people all over the country about weight loss and health and is working on a book of her own.

"I'm just a normal person who went through an extraordinary journey—one that happened to be on national television," says Ali. "But the important thing is I want people to understand that they deserve to have what I have, too—they deserve to have their best possible lives. I want to lead by example, and I'm an example of what it looks like to believe in yourself. If you can believe it, you can be it."

Ali says she finds it especially important to send the message to women that they deserve to put their health first.

"When did it become okay to give your time to every-one but yourself?" she says. "Women tend to nurture on so many different levels for so many people that they often forget to take care of themselves.

"It's so important to check in with yourself, no matter how busy you are—to ask yourself what you need to live a happy life. Finding the time for exercise can be a challenge, but you can start with small steps—finding ways to incorporate more activity into your day. You don't have to go to the gym. You can ride bikes with your husband in the morning before work, take your dog for a walk, run the perimeter of the soccer field while your kids are at practice."

Ali says she still pinches herself in disbelief that her life has turned 180 degrees from what it was in October of 2007, when she and her mom, Bette-Sue Burklund, first set foot on the ranch. Even though they were eliminated just 4 weeks into their stay, Ali never gave up; she kept working hard to lose weight at home. It's that hard work that earned her the right to return to the ranch later that season and, eventually, claim the grand prize.

Today she loves living a healthy lifestyle and helping others do the same. "Being comfortable with myself, finding balance, taking care of myself—it's liberation in the truest sense."

Ali's Simple Swaps

■ Swap fattening sauces for fresh salsa. "In the past, I always thought that healthy food had to taste bland, but on the ranch I had to get past my 'little girl' tastebuds and quit thinking that I hated tomatoes and onions or other veggies. So I turned to salsa for flavor I liked until I was comfortable trying more vegetables."

■ Swap a dinner date for an active date. Instead of being trapped in an unhealthy food environ-ment, offer your hostess a platter of healthy, homemade snacks. "Bring a trio of flavors of hummus and a variety of veggies. Everyone will love it, and you'll feel comfortable snacking with the rest of them."

■ Swap self-consciousness for self-belief. "I remember when I was home after being eliminated, and I was running on the treadmill. I told my brother how embarrassing it was because everything was jiggling, and he said, 'If it's moving, it's losing.' I loved that!"

■ Swap shyness for trying new things. "Don't be shy. I like to join group fitness classes that allow me to push myself to levels I wouldn't necessar-ily reach on my own. They give me opportunities to push through the uncomfortable."

Everyone Struggles with Something

Season 6 Winner

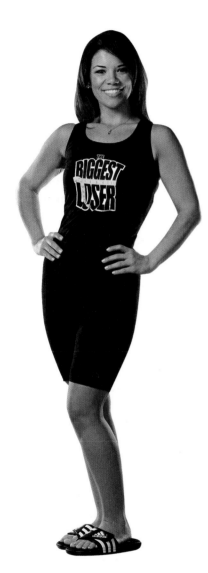

Starting weight: 242 pounds

Height: 5'3"

Home: Dallas

Finale weight: 132 pounds

Weight today: "That's between me and my bathroom scale."

Michelle Aguilar is not a big believer in numbers, especially when it comes to weight. "There is not a perfect number," she says. "You're perfect when you're feeling your best. My number is not your number. My weight doesn't define me. What do I weigh today? I'm not really sure."

In case you think she's trying to cover up some awful truth, think again. What she will reveal is that she wore a size 2/4 for the Season 6 finale—at which she won the grand prize and became the second female *Biggest Loser*. When Michelle got married about 6 months later, her wedding dress was a size 6. Clearly, she has nothing to hide!

Michelle learned the hard way that letting go of control was her ticket to success. She arrived at the ranch with her mom and teammate, Renee, and began the tough emotional work of coming to terms with her parents' divorce. "When I stopped trying to smile all the time and just let myself fall apart, that's when the show became successful for me. I realized that everyone struggles with something. They may not struggle with weight, but struggle is a part of everyone's journey, and that's what connects me to people."

Unlike some contestants who struggle with the prospect of going home, Michelle says she was prepared to leave the ranch. "We all have to go home sometime," she says. "And Jillian and I spent a lot of time talking about what that would be like, so that helped set me up for going home. I had tools, and now I was going to use them."

Michelle says she doesn't count calories anymore, but she does keep a running tab in her head regarding what she eats. "I plan for what I'm going to eat each day," she explains. "I think about it." She also sticks to a consistent workout routine of cardio and strength training 3 days a week for about 2 hours a session. "I exercise mostly in the gym. I'm not really an outdoor kind of girl," she laughs. "But the gym feels like a second home to me now. I'm not intimated by it anymore."

She's also banished guilt, or at least banished getting stuck in a guilt rut. "That's been one of my biggest hurdles. Now, instead of letting one bad day turn into a bad 6 years, I just start the next day with a lighter breakfast and a workout."

Michelle says she's also continuing the healing process regarding her parents' divorce. "When I wanted to quit the show at one point, my mom said, 'Listen, I'm going to love you no matter what you do; my love for you doesn't change.' For a mom to tell a daughter that speaks volumes. We all want to be supported. Plus, she understands the weight-loss journey, the struggles I've faced. She understands the big picture, and not everyone does."

What Michelle knows today is that she has embraced changes for a lifetime. "Before, if someone would just tell me how many steps I had to take to lose the weight and get it over with, that's what I wanted. Now, I understand that what I do to stay healthy is an ongoing, daily part of my life."

Michelle's Simple Swaps

- Swap hiding for seeking. "In order to be successful from the inside out, you have to face your demons. On the show, I had to break down and fall apart and do a lot of digging emotionally to come out on the other side."
- Swap caving in for grit and determination. "Remind yourself how far you've come. Put slips into perspective. You've been through worse than this. Apply that same grit and determination to get back on your feet tomorrow."
- Swap isolation for a phone call. "If I'm having a hard moment and struggling to get perspective on a situation, I call my sister and my mom, and they often jolt me back to reality."
- Swap the big picture for the small one. "It's making little changes every day that's going to lead to a healthier lifestyle in the long term. Today, drink more water. Tomorrow, take a walk."
- Swap store-bought lemonade for homemade limeade. "I used to drink tons of lemonade that had a lot of sugar. Today, I take sparkling water, add some sugar substitute, and squeeze a little lime into it. It gives me a break from drinking water; it's something different and refreshing."
- Swap big bags for little bags. "If you buy a big bag of chips, portion out servings in little baggies instead of eating blindly from the big bag. That way you know the exact calorie count."

Fueled by Competition

Hebe Salana

Starting weight: 294 pounds

Height: 5'10"

Home: Raleigh, North Carolina

Finale weight: 156 pounds

Weight today: 173 to 188 pounds

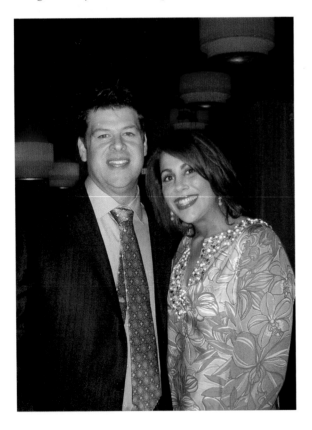

Ed Brantley

Starting weight: 335 pounds

Height: 6'3"

Home: Raleigh, North Carolina

Finale weight: 196 pounds

Weight today: Low 220s

Heba Salama confesses that she weighed her finale weight for "about 5 minutes." Season 6's $100,000 at-home prizewinner for the greatest percentage of weight lost off the ranch says some women like to be "thin-thin, but I'm not one of them." She's found a weight range that works for her and where she feels best. She and her husband, Ed Brantley, who were a team on the show, are fully embracing their new active lifestyle. In fact, they say they were happy to return to real life after *The Biggest Loser*.

Heba and Ed have found a passion for training for and participating in triathlons. Recently, they joined fellow *Biggest Loser* alumni in San Francisco for one such event. Heba says she was especially proud of Ed, who only recently learned how to swim, completing the swim in San Francisco Bay in 42 minutes! He was only 5 minutes behind her and 10 minutes behind Season 5 *Biggest Loser* Ali Vincent, a former nationally ranked swimmer.

Ed, a catering chef, runs a healthy cooking business, and together he and Heba conduct wellness seminars and offer free childhood obesity talks in North Carolina. "I love that I'm able to take the value of all the diet and exercise training that I received on the show and offer it to others for nothing," says Heba.

She says that when they speak to audiences of kids, she and Ed "stay away from the word *diet*. Girls especially can get fixated on that word, and we'd rather talk to them about being active and learning about calories." Heba and Ed also urge kids and their parents to turn off the TV and get rid of as much processed food as possible in their kitchens.

When it comes to fast food, Heba and Ed say a grilled chicken sandwich takes no longer to order than a cheeseburger. You can at least make a healthier choice with a leaner protein option. And they urge clients to start writing down everything they eat in a day before even counting calories, just to build an awareness of how much they consume. "Do that for 3 days," they say, "and commit to 30 minutes of movement for the first 30 days."

Heba and Ed have enjoyed getting to know and spend time with other past *Biggest Loser* contestants, including Daniel Wright, who also lives in North Carolina, and Amy Cremen, who was recently planning a visit. "We're going to go whitewater rafting together, something we never would have done before!" says Heba.

Heba and Ed's Simple Swaps

■ Swap microwave popcorn for popping your own kernels. Heba and Ed buy plain kernels and pop it on the stovetop—they swear it tastes better. They can control the sodium, and if they're in the mood for something sweet, they drizzle on a tiny bit of honey.

■ Swap date night out for date night in. Instead of going out to a fancy, calorie-rich dinner on a Saturday night, Heba and Ed try to do something active that they both enjoy, such as going to the pool or hiking or biking.

■ Swap thinking it's going to be easy for accepting that it's not. "I have to remind myself where I came from," says Heba. That was almost 300 pounds and a size 24 dress. "The daily struggle is still there. Every meal is a choice."

■ Swap a tired workout for an inspired one. Heba says when they feel their motivation flagging on the treadmill at home, they just pop in a Season 6 DVD. "Watching ourselves do those last-chance workouts is totally motivating," says Heba. Try using something that inspires you to keep going, too, whether it's fast-paced music or a DVD of *Rocky*!

Saying "I Do" to Life

Nicole

Starting weight: 269 pounds

Height: 5'7"

Home: Brooklyn, New York

Finale weight: 146 pounds

Weight today: She doesn't get on the scale.

Damien

Starting weight: 381 pounds

Height: 5'11"

Home: Brooklyn, New York

Finale weight: 245 pounds

Weight today: 241 pounds

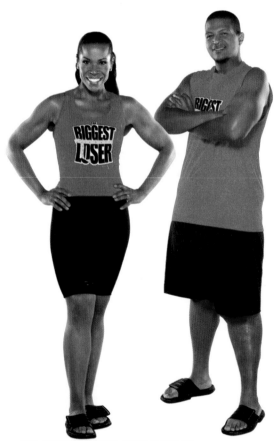

Few people have trod a more winding path to the altar than Damien and Nicole Gurganious. They got engaged in November 2007. Then they decided to try out for *The Biggest Loser*. After coming close but not being cast for Season 6 in early 2008, they went ahead and set a wedding date for November. A few months before her anticipated wedding date, Nicole bought her size 24 wedding dress. She was happy, but sad. Days later, a casting director for the show called and asked if they wanted to try out for Season 7. So they did, and this time . . . they ended up as contestants. After a flurry of frantic phone calls to caterers and relatives, the wedding was postponed.

Just days into Season 7, there was a surprise twist. The contestants found out that half of them would go home for 30 days before returning to the ranch for a chance to stay. The couple decided that Damien would stay and Nicole would head back to Brooklyn to continue her weight-loss journey there.

"When I went home those first 30 days," said Nicole, "I knew I was going to lose the weight. I could not let Damien down, or myself, for that matter. I knew this show was going to change my life." She went to the shop where she'd bought her wedding dress and asked if she could return it. Less than a year later, a stunning Nicole walked down the aisle wearing a size 8 wedding dress.

Nicole and Damien lost most of their weight during their time away from the ranch, which they now see as a blessing. "We got to come home and do this together and figure it out," says Nicole. "We know how to lose the weight right here." For Damien, having his wife and weight-loss partner in the same person is invaluable. "My wife was on the show with me," he says. "She's my account-ability partner and staring at me every day. It's a blessing and a curse," he laughs.

These days, Nicole prefers not to weigh herself regularly."I just don't like being traumatized by a number. So I have a suit that I use to gauge my weight. If it gets tight, I do something about it. If it fits, I'm fine."

Now this happy, fit couple is looking forward to living an active life together. Nicole has become a runner and even participated in a triathlon the week before her wedding. "I'm going to have finish lines in my life forever. Before, I wouldn't even run for the bus," says Nicole. "We can't wait to go to an amusement park. We can fit in the seats! And kayaking. Before, we couldn't fit in a kayak!"

Nicole and Damien's Simple Swaps

- Swap giving in for daily accountability. "I know some days I can be one triple cheeseburger away from going back to my old ways. It's important that I follow my workout and eating plan every single day," says Nicole.
- Swap a straw for a spoon. "I love to blend frozen berries to a smoothie consistency and eat it with a spoon. It's more satisfying than sipping through a straw," says Nicole.
- Swap food rewards for nonfood rewards. "I love to read," says Damien. "So after I take off my next 15 pounds, I'm buying an e-reader! It's my new motivation."
- Swap mountains for molehills. "Break down your weight-loss goal into weekly goals," says Damien. "If you need to lose 80 pounds, shoot for 2 pounds a week. That way it's a feasible, obtainable goal."

Paying It Forward One Child at a Time

UPDATE: Helen Phillips Season 7 Winner

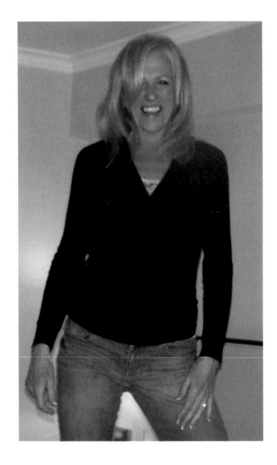

Starting weight: 257 pounds

Height: 5'6"

Home: Sterling Heights, Michigan

Finale weight: 117 pounds

Weight today: 129 pounds

When Helen Phillips was at her son's school gym getting in a workout before the Season 7 finale, she noticed that a lot of the kids around her were overweight. "There I was at the age of 48, and I was outperforming them," she says. "Then I'd watch them go line up for cafeteria food that was bad for them. Plus, I was in a depression when I was overweight, and I could see it happening to them. If I could change, I knew they could, too." It was then that she vowed to come back after *The Biggest Loser* and start doing what she could to address the nation's childhood obesity problem.

Today Helen is working with the Henry Ford Hospital as well as local restaurants and schools to come up with healthy lifestyle changes involving diet, exercise, and mental health for kids and their parents. Convincing overweight kids' parents—who are often overweight themselves—to make changes can be a challenge, she says. "It's sometimes tough to get the parents out of the habit of picking up fast food for dinner because it's hard to make the time to cook. Yeah, it's hard. I know that. But 'easier' doesn't mean 'better.'" As Helen points out, the "easier" can lead to diabetes and other obesity-related diseases for their kids.

Getting the kids to start moving is the next part of the challenge. "Kids come home, grab a snack (often junk food), and then sit in front of the TV or computer. Parents really need to make some changes to that routine. Get your kids to go out for a bike ride with you, or walk around the block together. That's all it takes to start making changes."

Helen learned about compromise and balance with her own teenage son, Alex. When she was fresh off the ranch, she had the zeal of a healthy lifestyle convert. "My freezer used to be full of pizzas and my fridge full of sodas. I cleaned all that out. Alex was on board, but he's 17. He wants a cheeseburger sometimes. Now, instead of freaking out about it, I know that he eats more of his meals at home and that they're healthy. I don't freak out about the occasional cheeseburger."

Helen has reached a comfortable weight of 129 pounds after her finale weight of 117. Like most contestants, she's allowed herself to find the weight where she feels healthiest and happiest. She's not worried about backsliding to her old ways. "I feel too good to go back to feeling bad again. I got it on the ranch. I know what it takes to stay healthy.

Now I just want to share that knowledge and hope with as many other families as possible. It's my time to pay it forward to the community."

Helen's Simple Swaps

- Swap grilled burgers for grilled portobello mushrooms. "I sauté veggies and put them on top of the mushrooms with some low-fat mozzarella and shrimp or grilled chicken."
- Swap cakes and pastries for fruit. "I went to a family reunion recently, and instead of tables groaning with cakes, we had one low-fat cake and lots of fresh fruit."
- Swap an obstacle for a creative solution. "When I left the ranch, I missed hiking in the hills. We don't exactly have hills in my subdivision, so I bought a canoe and now go canoeing up north!"
- Swap a grocery store trip for a visit to an ethnic market. "I took my son to a big outdoor Middle Eastern market, and we came home with all sorts of vegetables for a big stir-fry, plus eggplant for grilling and then mashing up into a puree."
- Swap walking one block for walking two blocks. "Just increase your distance a little each day. Do it gradually. Every day, take an extra step. That's all it takes to lead to big changes down the road."

2

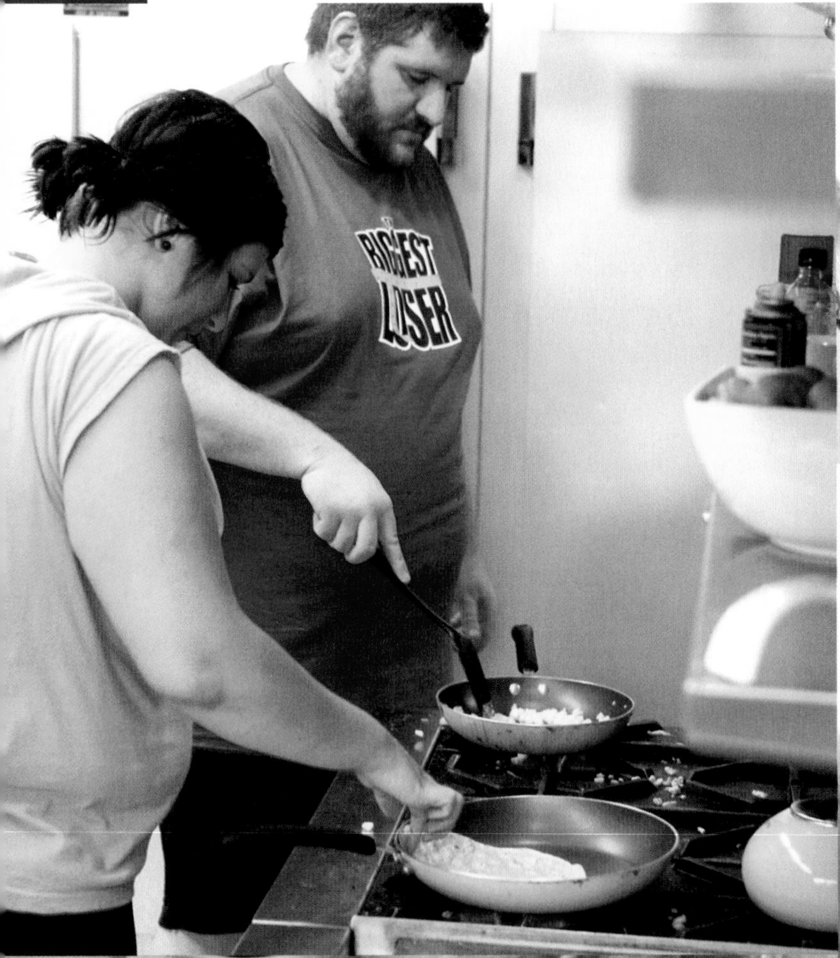

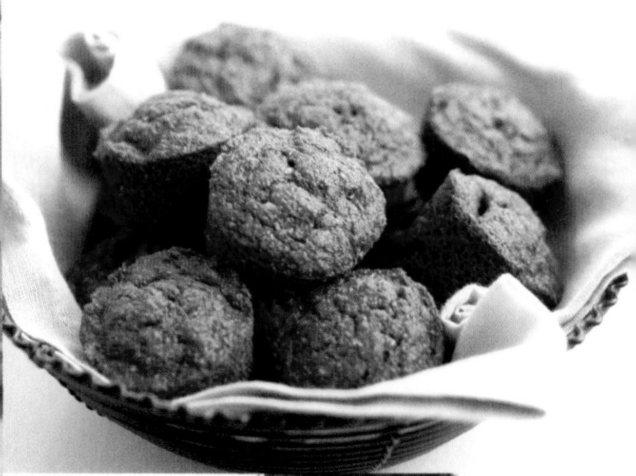

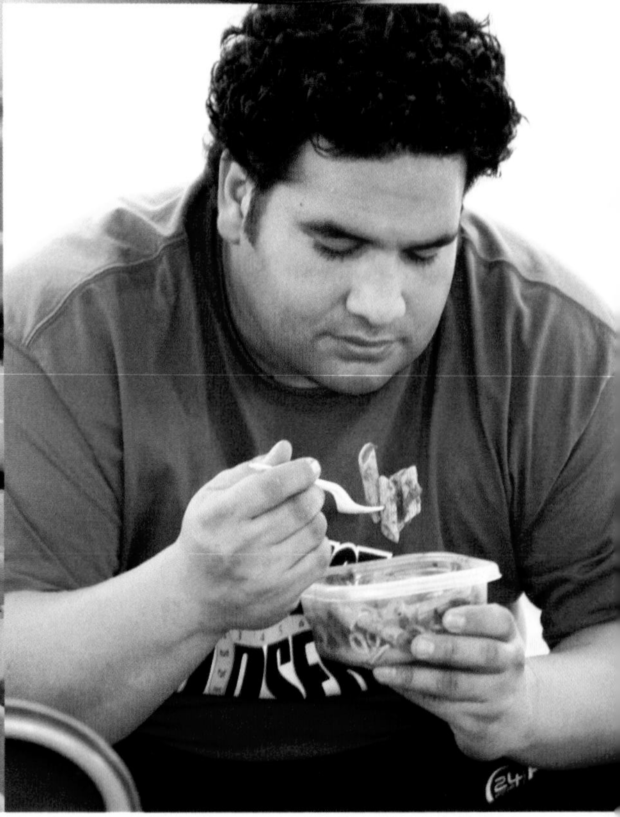

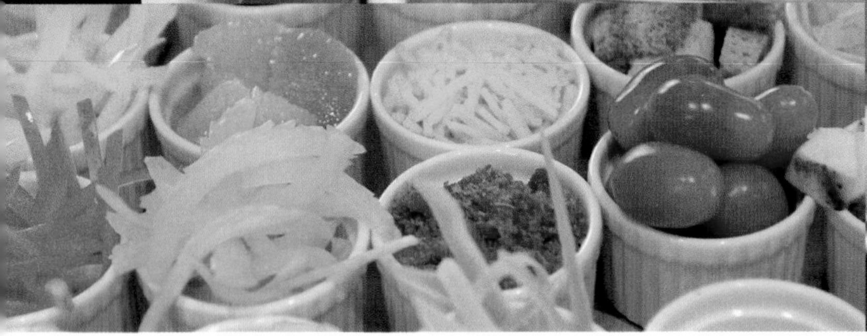

Calories: You Can Count on Them

As you probably know by now, when it comes to weight loss, there are no miracle solutions or magic pills. Getting your body fit and healthy all boils down to one thing: calories in, calories out. In order to lose weight, you must burn more calories than you consume. Obesity is caused by the opposite of this—consuming more calories than your body burns. As Season 7 finalist Tara Costa says, "You don't get to 294 pounds by accident."

When most contestants arrive at the ranch, they have no idea how many calories they've been eating, let alone how many calories they *should* be eating. In the pages that follow, you'll learn what they learn on campus: how to calculate a daily calorie budget based on your individual needs and weight-loss goals, how to distribute those calories throughout the day, and from what kinds of foods those calories should come.

Not all calories are created equal. While it's important to stay within your daily calorie budget and be mindful of the number you're consuming, it's just as important to be careful about the sources of those calories.

Medical Tip from DR. ROBERT HUIZENGA, *The Biggest Loser* Doctor

It's clear that the contestants on *The Biggest Loser* need to get healthy. How do you know if *you're* heading down a dangerous fat road? If you've put on 15 to 20 pounds since your early twenties, or if you've moved up two or more clothing sizes (or notches on your belt), it's time to make a change. Weight gain that is the result of an increase in body fat elevates your risk of heart disease and stroke.

Some calories will fuel your workouts, help you feel full and satisfied, and help boost your body's immune system and protect you from disease. Other calories don't really provide any benefits— in fact, they can actually make you feel tired, sluggish, and hungrier than you were *before* you ate.

So if you're going to lose weight and get healthy, the first thing you need to do is understand how to fuel your body the right way. On *The Biggest Loser* eating plan, each day you'll aim to eat at least four servings of vegetables and fruits; 30 percent of your calories will come from lean proteins; you'll choose two servings of whole-grain carbohydrates; no more than 25 percent of your daily calories will come from fat; and your sodium intake will be limited to 2,400 milligrams a day or less. When your body is given the nutrients and energy it needs, not only will you lose weight, you'll also *feel better* than ever.

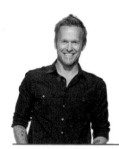

$ BUDGET TIP $
Portions That Make Cents
Another added benefit to measuring out your portions? You'll probably end up with less food waste. How many times have you poured the milk from the bottom of your cereal bowl down the drain when you've finished eating? Using exact portions saves you calories *and* money.

What Is a Calorie?

A calorie is a measurement of how much energy food provides after it has been consumed. Your body needs energy to fuel physical activity as well as all metabolic processes, from maintaining your heartbeat and growing hair to healing a broken bone and building lean muscle mass. Only four components of the food you eat supply calories: protein and carbohydrates (4 calories per gram), alcohol (7 calories per gram), and fat (9 calories per gram). Vitamins, minerals, fiber, and water do not supply calories.

The Biggest Loser eating plan helps you determine the exact calorie intake (your calorie budget)

Trainer Tip: BOB HARPER

Keep a food journal! Write down every calorie you consume. It will hold you accountable for all your food and beverage choices. It's been reported that keeping a food journal can even double your weight loss. Write everything down, and use *The Biggest Loser Calorie Counter* to help you determine the caloric value of each item. As long as you've burned more calories than you've taken in, you'll lose weight.

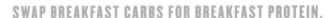

SWAP BREAKFAST CARBS FOR BREAKFAST PROTEIN.

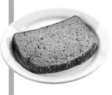

Don't forget that you need protein with every meal and snack. If you're going to have cereal for breakfast, be sure to pair it with skim milk; if you're going to eat toast, pair it with an egg. Combining carbs and protein is a great way to fuel up for the day ahead.

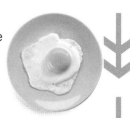

you require to meet your individual weight-loss goals. If you weigh 150 pounds or more, the simple formula on the following page, created by *The Biggest Loser* experts, will help you calculate how many calories you need each day. If you weigh less than 150 pounds, talk to your doctor about a calorie budget based on your individual weight-loss needs.

Your present weight × 7 =
Your daily calorie needs for weight loss

Your calorie budget should *never* be static; in fact, it's a moving target. As you lose weight on this plan—and you will—you'll need to continually reassess and reduce your calorie budget in order to keep losing weight at a good pace and break through plateaus.

It's important to keep in mind that everyone is different, and we all burn different numbers of calories at different rates. So if you and your spouse or friend follow this eating plan together,

one of you might lose weight at a different rate—faster or slower—than the other. Just like the contestants on *The Biggest Loser,* you may have huge losses one week, yet stay the same or even go up a pound the next.

For both men and women, losing weight is a process. It's never a straight, narrow path to your goal. There will be ups and downs and even plateaus, but that's perfectly normal. Weight loss is always rapid

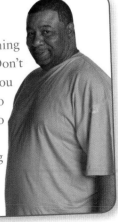

Mo DeWalt, Season 8

You can do anything. Anything is possible. I've been there. Don't just sit back. Become who you need to be, who you want to be. Learn how to eat, how to exercise. Do what you have to do. It starts with thinking that you can be a *Biggest Loser,* too.

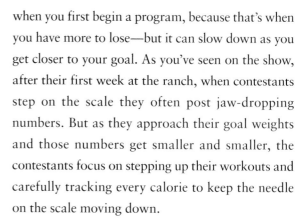

SWAP BOXES AND WRAPPERS FOR LEAVES AND PEELS.

Choosing more fresh produce and less processed food is central to *The Biggest Loser* eating plan. When you go to the grocery store, shop the perimeter first and load up on fruits and vegetables before hitting the aisles that contain boxed or canned goods.

SWAP YOUR CANDY DISH FOR A BASKET.

Reach for an apple, not an M&M. Keep a basket on your kitchen table or on your desk at work and fill it up with fresh fruit like apples, oranges, pears, and bananas each week. When healthy food is within arm's reach, you're much more likely to make a good snack choice the next time hunger strikes.

SWAP CALORIES FOR WATER.

Foods that are high in water content tend to be low in calorie density. That means they'll fill you up without a high number of calories. Swap more high-water foods such as broccoli, mushrooms, lettuces, spinach, tomatoes, apples, berries, and watermelon into your diet and feel fuller while spending less of your calorie budget.

when you first begin a program, because that's when you have more to lose—but it can slow down as you get closer to your goal. As you've seen on the show, after their first week at the ranch, when contestants step on the scale they often post jaw-dropping numbers. But as they approach their goal weights and those numbers get smaller and smaller, the contestants focus on stepping up their workouts and carefully tracking every calorie to keep the needle on the scale moving down.

Age is another factor in weight loss. Our muscles burn a lot of calories each day—about 10 times as many as our fat tissue does. But muscles shrink with age, which means we have a natural tendency to burn fewer calories as we get older. So as our muscle decreases, our body fat increases. While you may lose weight more slowly as you get older, don't let that hold you back from your goals. Season 7's Helen Phillips became *The Biggest Loser* at the age

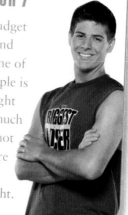

Mike Morelli, Season 7

I budget my food like I budget money. Just have a plan and have structure, because one of the hardest things for people is being accountable. In weight loss, you can work out as much as you want, but if you're not accountable for what you're eating or if you're eating poorly, you won't lose weight.

of 48, beating out much younger contestants for the grand prize. And Season 7 castmate Jerry Hayes won the at-home prize for the highest percentage of weight loss at the age of 63! As Jerry said in the weeks before the finale, "Before *The Biggest Loser*, I sold myself short. The more I do, the stronger my heart gets; the stronger my body gets. I'm just amazed." Helen and Jerry are living proof that you can get healthy at any age!

Allocating Your Calories

Now that you've determined your calorie budget, the next step is learning how to follow it. How do you divide up your calories throughout the day?

First you'll need to familiarize yourself with serving sizes. It's important to weigh and measure food so that you know exactly how many calories you're consuming each day. It's useful to have the following tools (many of which you may already own) to help you measure your serving sizes:

$ BUDGET TIP $

Calling All Calories!

These days, most cell phones and other mobile devices contain calculator features—check the functions on your device before running out to buy a calculator. Not only will you save money, but you'll also save space in your pocket or purse by needing to carry only one device!

- Liquid measuring cup (2-cup capacity)
- Set of dry measuring cups (includes 1-cup, ½-cup, ⅓-cup, and ¼-cup sizes)
- Measuring spoons (1 tablespoon, 1 teaspoon, ½ teaspoon, and ¼ teaspoon)
- Food scale
- Calculator

Be sure that your food scale measures grams. (A gram is very small, about $\frac{1}{28}$ of an ounce.) Most of your weight measurements will be in ounces, but certain foods, such as nuts, are very concentrated in calories, so you may need to measure your portion size in grams. There are a wide range of food scales

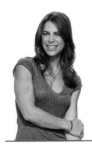

Trainer Tip: JILLIAN MICHAELS

Remove tempting foods from your home or from the table (like the bread basket!) when eating out. Willpower is a muscle you need to exercise, but removing temptation before it can get to you is a smart strategy.

available these days. To purchase the same scale the contestants use at the ranch, go to BiggestLoser.com. While *The Biggest Loser* scale and many other scales include a helpful feature that counts calories, I recommend that you also continue to count calories the old-fashioned way. You can never be too careful when it comes to tracking your calorie budget.

Getting Started

Your portion sizes are probably about to get smaller—and soon, your clothes will, too! You can still enjoy cereal in your favorite bowl each morning. But instead of just opening up the box and pouring in as much as you want, measure out a serving size (based on your calorie budget) and put only that much cereal in your bowl. Then do the same with your milk—measure it and pour it into the bowl instead of just dousing your cereal with milk straight from the carton. Do you notice a difference between how this breakfast looks and your usual bowl of cereal? Take a mental note. Though it's best to keep measuring until you get used to it, eventually the goal is to be able to eyeball serving sizes.

When it comes to cooking, food should be weighed or measured *after* cooking. For example, 4 ounces of boneless, skinless chicken breast has around 140 calories when raw. When it's cooked, it'll weigh closer to 3 ounces. That's because it loses water during the cooking process, and the calories become more concentrated. The same holds true for vegetables and other cooked foods. Dry cereals or grains, on the other hand, may be only a few tablespoons per serving initially, but once you add water and cook them, their volume may double or triple.

Over time, you'll know what's just right for you,

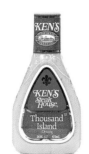

SWAP UNHEALTHY FATS FOR FLAVORFUL OILS.

While it's true that fats have more calories than protein and carbs do, good fats play an important role in a healthy eating plan. When choosing oils to add to your salad, skip the premade dressings that can contain trans fat and opt for a tablespoon of sesame oil, extra virgin olive oil, or walnut oil. You'll get more flavor (and nutrient) bang for the same calorie buck.

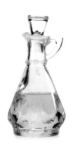

whether you're plating a meal in your own kitchen or deciding how much of an entrée to eat in a restaurant (and how much of it to wrap up and take home!). If you're not accustomed to spending time in the kitchen, the conversion table below may be helpful to you.

Remember that an ounce of *weight* is not the same as a *fluid* ounce. For some of the foods listed on pages 36 to 39, you'll use a measuring cup to count the calories in a serving. For other foods, you'll measure your calories in ounces or grams. This is why you'll require a scale and measuring cups and spoons to get started.

Dina Mercado, Season 8

The quality of the calories I've learned to eat on the ranch is so different from what I used to eat. Before, I'd try to fill myself up with burgers and fries and all those empty calories, and it was never enough. I was eating thousands of empty calories and not feeling full. Now I feel satisfied on so much less.

CONVERSION TABLE FOR MEASURING PORTION SIZES

TEASPOONS	TABLESPOONS	CUPS	PINTS, QUARTS, GALLONS	FLUID OUNCES	MILLILITERS
¼ teaspoon					1 milliliter
½ teaspoon					2 milliliters
1 teaspoon	⅓ tablespoon				5 milliliters
3 teaspoons	1 tablespoon	¹⁄₁₆ cup		½ ounce	15 milliliters
6 teaspoons	2 tablespoons	⅛ cup		1 ounce	30 milliliters
12 teaspoons	4 tablespoons	¼ cup		2 ounces	60 milliliters
16 teaspoons	5⅓ tablespoons	⅓ cup		2½ ounces	75 milliliters
24 teaspoons	8 tablespoons	½ cup		4 ounces	125 milliliters
32 teaspoons	10⅔ tablespoons	⅔ cup		5 ounces	150 milliliters
36 teaspoons	12 tablespoons	¾ cup		6 ounces	175 milliliters
48 teaspoons	16 tablespoons	1 cup	½ pint	8 ounces	237 milliliters
		2 cups	1 pint	16 ounces	473 milliliters
		3 cups		24 ounces	710 milliliters
		4 cups	1 quart	32 ounces	946 milliliters
		8 cups	½ gallon	64 ounces	
		16 cups	1 gallon	128 ounces	

Your calculator will be an indispensable tool when it comes to measuring food portions. Sometimes the portion size you want may be different from the serving size provided in a recipe or on the packaging of a product. You may have to do a little math to adjust the portion of food you eat to stay within your calorie budget. This is great practice for life outside your kitchen, because you will rarely find your ideal portion sizes when you dine out.

Food Journal

Keeping a food journal is paramount to a successful weight-loss plan. It will help you see what you're really eating (be honest!) and learn from your eating patterns. It's imperative to keep track of the number of calories you take in and burn off through exercise each day. Keep a notebook and a pen with you at all times just for this purpose. Take notes throughout the day, because it's easy to forget an unplanned snack or a "taste" you had while cooking. Create a routine: Find a favorite place and time to record your intake and workouts in your journal, and stick to it.

Keeping a food journal will require you to become an expert at reading food labels and Nutrition Facts panels. When you're shopping for healthy foods, labels can help you choose between similar products based on calorie and nutrient (such as fat, protein, or fiber) content.

The label at right is an example of what you'll find on the packaging of any item at your local supermarket. It contains a lot of information, but here are the parts you most need to pay attention to.

Serving size: This is the most important thing to note, because everything else on the label (calories, grams of fat, etc.) is based on this measurement. Just because a food label suggests a serving size doesn't mean that it's the right serving size for you.

Nutrition Facts

Serving Size
Servings Per Container

Amount Per Serving	
Calories 0	
Calories from Fat 0	
	% Daily Value*
Total Fat 0g	0%
Saturated Fat 0g	0%
Trans Fat 0g	
Cholesterol 0mg	0%
Sodium 0mg	0%
Total Carbohydrate 0g	0%
Dietary Fiber 0g	0%
Soluble Fiber 0g	0%
Insoluble Fiber 0g	0%
Sugars 0g	
Protein 0g	

Vitamin A 0%	•	Vitamin C 0%	
Calcium 0%	•	Iron 0%	
Phosphorus 0% • Magnesium 0%			

* Percent Daily Values are based on a 2,000 calo-rie diet. Your daily values may be higher or lower depending on your calorie needs:

		Calories:	2,000	2,500
Total Fat	Less than		0g	0g
Sat Fat	Less than		0g	0g
Cholesterol	Less than		0mg	0mg
Sodium	Less than		0mg	0mg
Potassium			0mg	0mg
Total Carbohydrate			0g	0g
Dietary Fiber			0g	0g

Calories per gram:
Fat 0 • Carbohydrate 0 • Protein 0

Abby Rike, Season 8

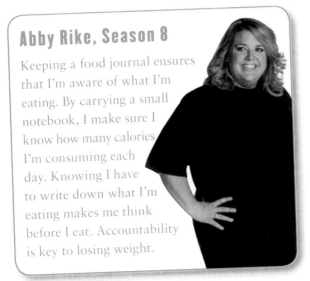

Keeping a food journal ensures that I'm aware of what I'm eating. By carrying a small notebook, I make sure I know how many calories I'm consuming each day. Knowing I have to write down what I'm eating makes me think before I eat. Accountability is key to losing weight.

Look at the calorie and fat content in light of the serving. If you need to, cut the serving size in half.

Calories: Be sure that the number of calories you record in your food journal reflects the number of

Danny Cahill, Season 8

Bad food is cheap and easy. For lunch, I used to eat 2,000 to 3,000 calories at one sitting. But now I have a calorie budget, and I'm eating food that's high in fiber and nutrient dense, and it's good stuff! When you eat fast food, you're getting all your calories from sugar and grease. It's not nutritious, it doesn't feed your body, and it makes you fat.

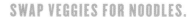

SWAP TAKEOUT FOR COOKING IN.

When you cut back on dining out and ordering in, you'll not only save money but undoubtedly save calories as well, since you know exactly what is going into the pan and how much to put on your plate. It might be less work to order a pizza—but it will result in more work at the gym!

SWAP SHOVELING FOR SAVORING.

Instead of inhaling the food on your plate, try to slow down, take smaller bites, and really taste your food. Eating more slowly not only is better for your digestion but also helps you enjoy your meal and allows your body to feel full before you've gone back for seconds.

SWAP VEGGIES FOR NOODLES.

It may sound counterintuitive, but the next time you're making a salad, instead of eating a mountain of lettuce, toss in ½ cup of cooked whole grain pasta. It will add texture, flavor, and, most important, satisfaction. Finish it off with a little protein in the form of chicken breast, hard-boiled egg whites, or turkey, and you've got a balanced meal.

SWAP WEIGHING YOURSELF EVERY DAY FOR WEIGHING YOUR FOOD EVERY DAY.

Try to get in the habit of weighing your food daily. After a while you'll be able to eyeball appropriate portion sizes, and food journaling will become easier. Weighing yourself is important for tracking your body's weight loss, but don't drive yourself crazy with daily weigh-ins—once a week is enough. Schedule a day and time to step on the scale each week and stick to it.

SWAP GIMMICKS FOR NUTRITION INFORMATION.

Don't fall for the language on the front of the package—some claims can be misleading (see page 37). Always read the nutrition labels on the side or back of the package and check the ingredient list. It's the only way to really know what you're eating.

Pay special attention to the numbers of calories on "light," reduced-fat, low-fat, and fat-free products. When the fat is removed from many recipes, salt or sugar is sometimes added to enhance the flavor. This can result in a fat-free or low-fat product that actually contains *more* calories than the regular version.

Saturated fat: Less than one-third of your daily grams of fat should come from saturated fats, which are derived mainly from animal products and are solid at room temperature (such as butter and shortening). Some plant oils, such as coconut oil and palm oil, are also saturated. The saturated fat from animal foods is the primary source of cholesterol.

Sodium: For most people, the daily recommended sodium intake is no more than 2,400 milligrams. Some of the foods you eat each day will have more, others less. Aim for an average of no more than 240 milligrams of sodium in each meal or snack.

servings you've eaten. If the label indicates that a serving is 1 cup and you ate 2 cups, you need to double the calories to match your double serving.

Total fat: The number of grams of fat in a product reflects the sum of three kinds of fat: saturated fat, polyunsaturated fat, and monounsaturated fat.

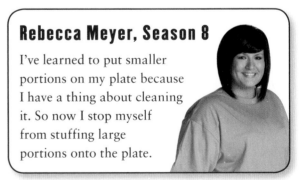

Rebecca Meyer, Season 8

I've learned to put smaller portions on my plate because I have a thing about cleaning it. So now I stop myself from stuffing large portions onto the plate.

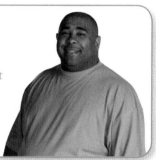

Total carbohydrate: This number is calculated by adding grams of complex carbohydrates plus grams of fiber plus grams of sugars. If the total carbohydrate number is more than double the amount of sugars, that means there are more "good carbs" than "bad carbs" in the food.

Dietary fiber: Fiber is found in plant foods but not in animal foods. Unless you're on a fiber-restricted diet, aim for at least 25 to 35 grams of fiber per day.

Sugars: The sugars in a food can be naturally occurring or added. Check the ingredient list to find out, and avoid eating foods that contain processed sugars, such as high-fructose corn syrup. The total grams of carbohydrates in a food serving should be more than twice the number of grams of sugar.

Protein: If a food has more than 9 grams of protein per serving, it's considered a high-protein food. It's important to eat foods that are high in protein when you're trying to lose weight, because protein is a great source of energy and helps you feel full.

Ingredient List

A product's ingredients are listed in order of decreasing weight. If the first few ingredients listed include any form of sugar (cane sugar, corn syrup, sucrose, and so on) or fats and oils, the food is probably not a good choice for weight loss. Also, look for products with a short list of ingredients you recognize. A long list of strange-sounding ingredients is always a red flag. Leave those products on the shelf at the grocery store—don't put them on the shelf of your pantry.

Now that you're a label expert, it's time to go shopping! The following pages contain lists of some common foods found in the cupboards of *The Biggest Loser* kitchen. These foods are all part of *The Biggest Loser* eating plan and are used by the contestants on the ranch. You don't need to go out and buy all these at once, but it's helpful to have a shopping list when you go to the store.

Fruit

Apples

Bananas

Blackberries

Blueberries

Cherries

Frozen fruit (all varieties except pineapple)

Goji berries, dried

Grapefruit

Lemons

Limes

Melons (all types)

Oranges, tangerines

Peaches

Plums

Raspberries

Strawberries

Vegetables

Artichokes

Asparagus

Avocados

Bell peppers (all colors)

Broccoli

Brussels sprouts

Carrots

Cauliflower

Celery

Cherry tomatoes

Cucumbers

Eggplant

Endive

Green beans

Jicama

Lettuce (all varieties)

Mushrooms

Onions

Spaghetti squash

Spinach (regular and baby)

Sprouts

Sweet potatoes

Tomatoes

Zucchini

Fresh Herbs and Seasonings

Basil

Cilantro

Garlic

Ginger

Italian parsley

Mint

Oregano

Thyme

Whole Grains

Brown rice

Brown rice pasta

Quinoa

Quinoa pasta

Steel-cut oatmeal

Whole grain breads

Whole grain cereals

Whole grain English muffins

Whole grain pasta

Whole grain tortillas

Beans and Legumes

Black beans

Chickpeas

Great Northern beans

Don't Judge a Food by Its Package

In addition to the nutrition labels and ingredient lists on the back of packaged foods, often you'll find bold promises on the front of these products—especially if the product is a "light" version of the original. These phrases are sometimes a little misleading. The list below decodes common health claims you'll find on many packaged goods.

- **Calorie free:** This designation means that the product must contain less than 5 calories per serving.

- **Low calorie:** This term means the food contains no more than 40 percent of the calories of the regular version.

- **Reduced calorie:** A reduced-calorie food contains at least 25 percent fewer calories than the regular version. Depending on how many calories the original version had, this doesn't necessarily guarantee that the food is low in calories.

- **Fat free:** A fat-free food can contain only 0.5 gram of fat (or less) per serving.

- **Low fat:** This phrase guarantees that there are 3 grams of fat (or less) per serving.

- **Light:** This term means a product has 50 percent less fat than its regular counterpart. Depending on how much fat the original product contains, this doesn't necessarily mean that the product is low in fat.

- **Reduced fat:** This term simply indicates that a product has 25 percent less fat than the regular version. Again, it doesn't necessarily mean that the food is low in fat.

- **High fiber:** This is a good term to watch for. It indicates that one serving has at least 5 grams of dietary fiber.

- **Good source of fiber:** This phrase guarantees that the food product has 2.5 to 4.9 grams of fiber per serving.

- **More or added fiber:** These claims mean that the product has at least 2.5 grams of fiber per serving—which doesn't necessarily mean it is "high fiber."

- **Low sodium:** These foods contain half the sodium of the original.

- **Sugar free:** This term guarantees that there is less than 0.5 gram of sugar per serving.

Lentils

Low-sodium prepared hummus

Red beans

Tofu

Unsweetened cocoa nibs

Nuts and Seeds

Almond butter

Dry roasted almonds

Flaxseeds or flax fiber

Hemp seed nuts

Peanut butter (unsalted)

Raw cashews

Raw pecans

Raw walnuts

Fish

Black cod

Halibut

Orange roughy

Red snapper

Scallops (wild)

Shrimp (wild)

Sole

Swordfish

Tilapia

Tuna (canned in water; no salt)

Tuna steaks (ahi and albacore)

Wild Alaskan salmon (not farm raised)

Poultry

Ground chicken (white meat)

Ground turkey breast (1% fat)

Skinless chicken breasts

Sliced turkey breast

Uncured, nitrite-free turkey bacon

Red Meat

Grass-fed lean ground beef, flank steak, and filet

Lean, low-sodium ham

Lean, low-sodium sliced roast beef cold cuts

Lean pork tenderloin

Alexandra White, Season 8

I just turned 20 years old, and I've been overweight my entire life. Between being in college and working, it was cafeteria food or fast food every day—whatever was quickest. Now I'm eating healthy foods, and it's fun to experiment with different combinations of foods that are good for me. They taste delicious and are surprisingly satisfying!

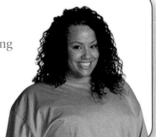

Eggs and Dairy

Egg whites

Fat-free and low-fat cottage cheese

Fat-free and low-fat (2%) Greek-style yogurt

Fat-free and 1% milk

Fat-free ricotta cheese

Lactaid fat-free milk

Low-fat and reduced-fat cheeses, including cream cheese and string cheese

Omega-3 whole eggs

Condiments, Oils, and Spices

Balsamic vinegar

Canola oil

Dried spices: Allspice, basil, black pepper, chili powder, cinnamon, crushed red pepper, curry, dill, oregano, rosemary, turmeric, etc.

Extra-virgin olive oil

Flaxseed oil

Fresh salsa

Galeos salad dressings (all flavors)

Horseradish

Low-sodium organic chicken broth or vegetable broth

Mrs. Dash sodium-free spice blends

Mustard (all kinds)

No-carbohydrate barbecue sauce and ketchup

No-sugar-added fruit spreads

No-sugar, low-sodium pasta sauce

Now Xylitol Plus packets

Rice wine vinegar

Stevia Extract 365

Tabasco sauce

Truvia

Beverages

The Biggest Loser Protein Powder

Black tea

Coffee

Green tea

Light vanilla soy milk

Unsweetened almond milk

Unsweetened cranberry juice

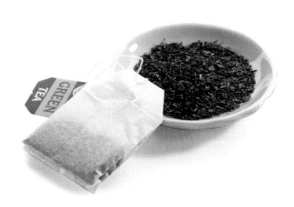

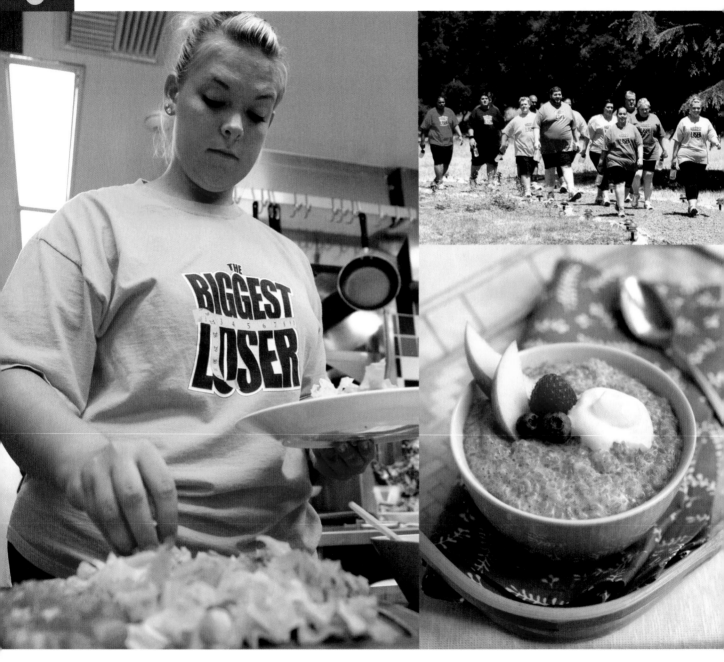

3

Planning Regular Meals and Snacks

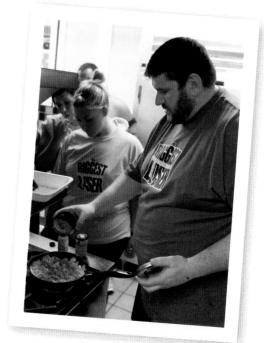

Trainer Jillian Michaels has a saying that's been passed down throughout the seasons of the show: "If you fail to plan, you plan to fail." As *The Biggest Loser* contestants quickly learn, planning is crucial to just about every aspect of weight loss. Planning meals, snacks, exercise sessions, even times to rest . . . preparation is essential to successful weight loss.

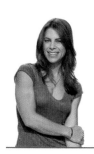

And the contestants' ability to plan is put to the test when they go home and live like the rest of us. Season 7 winner Helen Phillips remembers returning home to prepare for the finale. "I was a little disoriented," she said about being away from the ranch for the first time in months. There was no longer a gym just a few feet away from her bedroom

Trainer Tip: JILLIAN MICHAELS

Try eating about 85 percent of your meals at home. Research shows that you're more likely to overeat and consume more calories when you eat at restaurants.

door, and she didn't walk into a kitchen each day that was continually stocked with healthy groceries. She says she quickly realized: "Okay. I have to make a plan."

So she sat down and mapped out the next week. "I was always prepared," she said. "I always took food with me wherever I went so I wouldn't be hungry without a healthy snack nearby and wouldn't be tempted to go to the drive-thru. And I always stuck to my workout schedule." For Helen, making a plan and sticking to it was a way to achieve her goals and avoid temptation.

Nicole Brewer of Season 7 was on the ranch for only a couple of weeks but managed to lose 123 pounds all by herself back in Brooklyn, New York. The key to her success? "Writing down what I ate," she says. "I made sure I had healthy snacks on me at all times so I wasn't tempted by something I saw when I was walking down the street.

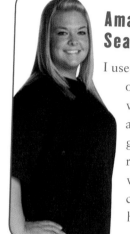

Amanda Arlauskas, Season 8

I used to snack way too much on horrible foods when I watched TV. I would take a box of cereal and a gallon of milk and keep refilling my bowl until I was full. Now I love baby carrots and hummus as healthier alternatives.

That's where the downfall would have been."

If you don't have a plan, you're rolling the dice with your weight-loss efforts. Season 8's Sean Algaier admits that he used to sit at his computer for 4 or 5 hours at a time without a meal or snack.

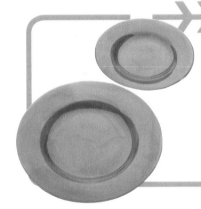

SWAP A KING-SIZE DINNER PLATE FOR A SALAD PLATE.

Whether you're dining out at a buffet or setting the table at home, chances are a smaller plate will hold all the food your calorie budget allows while helping you adapt to the portion sizes your body needs— not the sizes your eyes want!

"Then I would go out and try to find the fastest thing I could to satisfy this huge hunger," he said. "I would go to one of my favorite fast-food places and eat four cheeseburgers at time. Now I plan my mealtimes so I'm not tempted to eat something unhealthy at the last minute."

Dan Evans of Season 5 concurs with this and adds that he finds it essential to write down everything he eats. "Make sure you are totally conscious of what you're eating," he advises. "Otherwise, it's easy for your inner fat person to sneak back out."

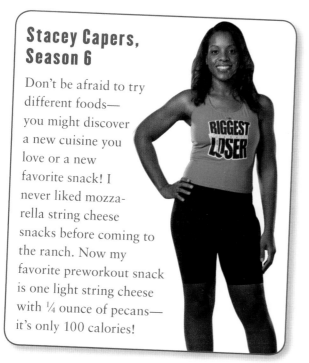

Stacey Capers, Season 6

Don't be afraid to try different foods—you might discover a new cuisine you love or a new favorite snack! I never liked mozzarella string cheese snacks before coming to the ranch. Now my favorite preworkout snack is one light string cheese with ¼ ounce of pecans—it's only 100 calories!

Don't Skip Meals

When contestants first arrive at *The Biggest Loser* ranch, they're often surprised to learn that one of the likely culprits in their weight gain is their tendency to skip meals (usually breakfast, lunch, or both). "Skipping meals was one of the worst habits I had prior to the show," says Season 8 contestant Shay Sorrells, who arrived at the ranch as the heaviest woman in the show's history, at 476 pounds. How can skipping meals lead to weight gain? It may not sound logical, but it's a fact: You need to feed your body at regular intervals to keep your metabolism charged. In fact, one recent study found that people who skipped meals during the day and consumed most of their calories at night exhibited

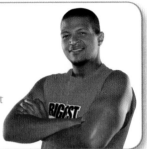

SWAP A LAST-MINUTE MENU CHOICE FOR A PLAN.

When you're going out to eat, it's important to have a plan. If you've never been to a restaurant before, look up its menu online so you know what to expect. Once you're there, ask for modifications, if needed, such as ordering the sauce on the side or requesting that your protein be grilled instead of fried. And just say no to the bread basket.

SWAP SNACK PACKS IN YOUR GROCERY CART FOR HEALTHY SNACK INGREDIENTS.

Buy fruit, vegetables, and other healthy snack options and keep them handy at all times. Unlike the empty calories in some "snack packs," these snacks will give you the fuel and nutrients you need to stay energized.

unhealthy changes in their metabolisms, similar to the unhealthy blood sugar levels observed in people with diabetes. The people who ate three regular meals throughout the day, on the other hand, consumed the same number of calories as the meal skippers but maintained healthy metabolisms.

"One of the biggest mistakes you can make is skipping meals," says Ron Morelli of Season 7. "I'm a creature of habit now. I eat every 4 hours." And Season 5 winner Ali Vincent says she always eats within half an hour of waking up to jump-start her metabolism. "Then I eat every 3 to 4 hours," she says. "I think this is just as important for me as exercise."

Listen to Hunger Cues

Another problem with skipping meals throughout the day is that when dinnertime finally rolls around, you're so hungry that it's easy to choose the wrong foods and, very often, eat too much of them. After all, who wants to nibble on carrot sticks when you're starving? It's hard not to be tempted by high-fat foods when you're very hungry. *Fat has more than twice as many calories as protein and carbohydrate.* It satisfies out-of-control hunger very quickly—and your body seems to know this. Fat often plays a big role in the unhealthy food choices made by people who skip meals.

The other problem with skipping meals is that when you wait too long to eat, you lose track of your body's natural hunger cues. You don't really know when you're hungry anymore—or when you're full. Most overeaters don't stop eating when they're no longer hungry and just satisfied—they don't feel as if they've finished a meal until they're uncomfortably stuffed. It's important to really get in tune with your body's hunger and satiety cues and feed it—or not—in response to its needs, not your cravings. You should never need to unbutton or unzip anything or lie down after a meal!

The scale below can help you identify and interpret your body's hunger cues.

If your hunger is anywhere from level 1 through 3, you should eat.

If you're at level 4, drink a glass of water, chew a piece of sugar-free gum, or do something else to distract yourself from thinking about food.

Hunger Scale

1. Famished or starving; you actually feel weak or light-headed. Don't allow yourself to get to this point.

2. Very hungry; you can't think of anything else but eating. You're cranky and irritable, and you can't concentrate.

3. Hungry; your stomach is growling or feels empty.

4. A little bit hungry; you're just starting to think about your next meal.

5. Satisfied; you're comfortable and aren't really thinking about food. You're alert and have a good energy level.

6. Fully satisfied; you've had enough to eat.

7. More than satisfied; you've had plenty to eat—maybe a little too much. Maybe you took a few extra bites.

8. Very full; you ate a little too much, but it tasted really good.

9. Uncomfortable; you're too full. You're bloated and tired, and you don't feel great.

10. Stuffed; you're uncomfortable and maybe even nauseated. Never allow yourself to get to this point.

SWAP YOUR COUCH FOR A TREADMILL.

Everyone has favorite TV shows they don't want to miss. Instead of watching them from your couch (within proximity of the fridge), head for the gym, where you can burn calories while catching up on the latest plot twists.

SWAP AN EXTRA HOUR AT THE OFFICE FOR AN EXTRA HOUR OF SLEEP.

Sure, this swap is easier said than done, especially when you're under pressure at work. But learning to say no and create boundaries is part of planning for a healthier life. Getting enough rest is crucial to your weight-loss efforts—don't sabotage yourself.

When you're trying to lose weight, you should try to stop eating when you reach level 5, but definitely no later than level 6. If you get to level 7, you've eaten too much. Anything above that is *way* too much and will sabotage your weight-loss efforts.

If you're not in the habit of eating regular meals throughout the day, try to set up a schedule that works for you. Successful *Biggest Loser* contestants learn over time that carefully planning three regular meals and two snacks each day is one of the most important elements of successful weight loss.

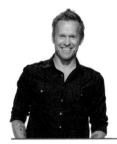
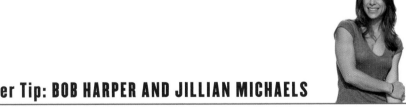

Trainer Tip: BOB HARPER AND JILLIAN MICHAELS

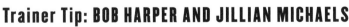

Don't go grocery shopping when you're hungry! Eat before you go, make a list, and stick to the items on your list.

Planning Your Budget

When I'm teaching the contestants at the ranch how to adjust to their new calorie budgets, I show them how to divide up their calories throughout the day to keep from getting hungry at any point. In the example below, I've used an 1,800-calorie budget, but your daily budget may be based on more or fewer calories. The equations remain the same.

Total daily calorie budget: 1,800

Divide your total daily calories by four to determine how many calories you can spend on meals and snacks.

$$1,800 \div 4 = 450$$

So for each meal—breakfast, lunch, and dinner—this person has a 450-calorie budget.

Now divide the remaining one-fourth of

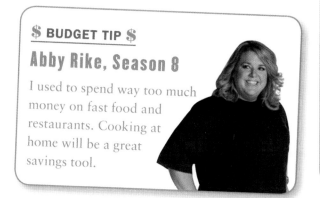

$ BUDGET TIP $

Abby Rike, Season 8

I used to spend way too much money on fast food and restaurants. Cooking at home will be a great savings tool.

SWAP A SECOND HELPING FOR A GOOD CONVERSATION.

Use your mealtime as an opportunity to unwind and reconnect with your family or friends. When you allow yourself a chance to digest dinner, you might realize that you aren't hungry anymore—and that connecting with loved ones is even better than dessert.

SWAP A DOUGHNUT FOR A PHONE CALL.

The next time a stress trigger hits in between meal or snack times, reach for the telephone instead of a comfort food. Talking to a friend or loved one is a much healthier way to deal with stress than letting yourself consume unwanted calories.

SWAP TV TIME FOR BROWN-BAGGING TIME.

Skip 10 minutes in front of the tube each night to assemble your snacks and meals for the next day. Not only will a few minutes enable you to stick to your plan, but you'll be surprised (and thrilled) at the money you'll save when you pack your food for the day instead of buying it already prepared.

your total daily calorie budget—in this case, 450—by two.

$$450 \div 2 = 225$$

So, for each of two daily snacks, this person has a 225-calorie budget.

This equation is just a starting point—use it to help you determine a distribution of calories throughout the day that keeps you satisfied. If you go to the gym in the morning, for example, and require a bigger breakfast to fuel your workout, feel free to shift your calorie intake toward the start of your day. You can move your calorie distribution around to suit your personal needs and schedule.

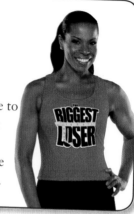

Nicole Brewer, Season 7

People say you have to choose to be happy. I believe in that. You have to choose to make the best out of every day. By planning ahead, I choose to be healthy and happy.

And if you're one of those people who prefer eating several small meals throughout the day, you can do that, too. Six 300-calorie meals throughout the day is certainly an option for someone on an 1,800-calorie budget. But, as Season 7's Blaine Cotter said, "There's something so satisfying about that feeling of fullness that follows a regular meal. I would miss it too much if I only had small meals!"

100-Calorie Snacks to Pack

These days, it's easy to find snacks in the supermarket that prominently display a calorie count of 100 (or lower) on the package. These portion-controlled treats can come in handy when you're in a pinch and don't want to blow your calorie budget on a

$ BUDGET TIP $
Daniel Wright, Seasons 7 and 8

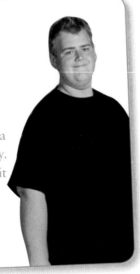

If I buy all my produce fresh, some of it will go bad in my fridge and be a complete waste of money. So I buy some of my fruit and veggies frozen. They're just as rich in vitamins and will keep longer in the freezer.

snack. Many of these products are healthy, though others don't contain nutrients like fiber and protein that will help you feel satisfied and full.

One of the cornerstones of *The Biggest Loser* food plan is that the quality of your calories is just as important as the quantity. With that in mind, here are some easy, nutritious snack options you can pack yourself that contain about 100 calories each.

- ½ cup of salsa and ⅓ cup of fat-free cottage cheese
- Half an apple, sliced and spread with 2 teaspoons of peanut butter
- Five or six almonds and ½ cup of grapes
- An 8-ounce carton of low-fat yogurt
- One hard-boiled egg
- 2 tablespoons of hummus with 1 cup of jicama slices
- About ½ cup of edamame
- One 3¼-inch pomegranate

SWAP A COFFEE BREAK FOR A WALK AND TALK.

If you work in an office, there's probably a time late in the afternoon when you and your coworkers gather for coffee, treats, and gossip. Save yourself calories (and money) by asking a colleague to join you for a 10-minute walk outside! Fresh air and exercise will give you more energy than a latte and a cookie.

Tracey Yukich, Season 8

Always sit at the table to eat. Don't snack while preparing your food. Eat slowly and enjoy your food. And when you're satisfied . . . *stop!* Don't overeat. Listen to your body.

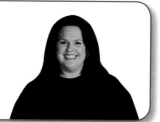

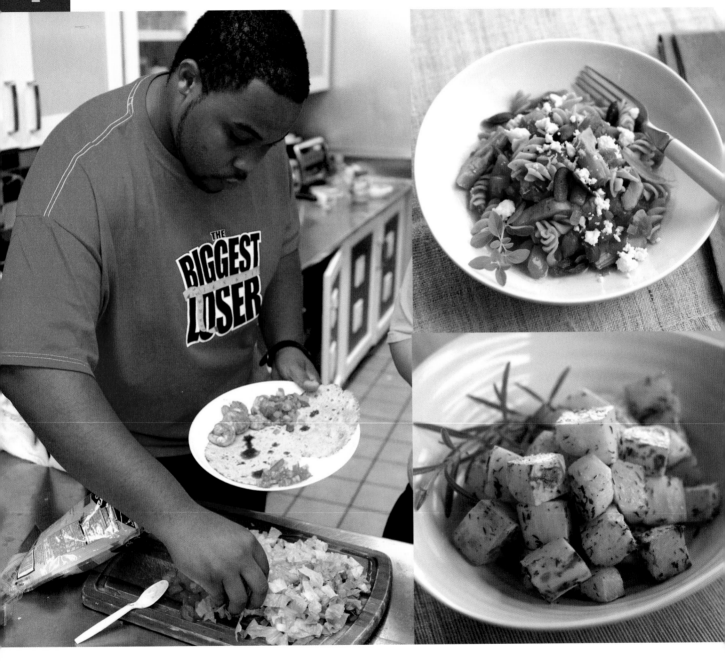

Eat Your Vegetables

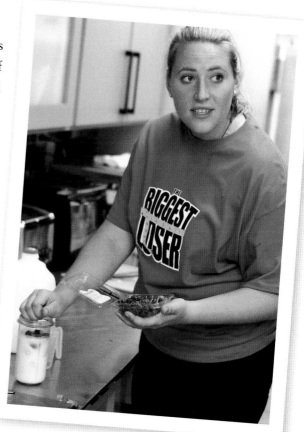

A lot of *Biggest Loser* contestants arrive at the ranch as serious fast-food junkies. In their preranch lives, most of their daily veggies came from whatever was sandwiched between a bun, snuggled next to a quarter pound of meat. When I sit down with them for their first nutrition consultation, they're disappointed to learn that lettuce, pickles, and ketchup don't satisfy their daily vegetable needs.

But fruits and vegetables are what's going to fill them up and keep them energized all day long. That's because fruits and vegetables are important sources of fiber. Fiber plays several key roles in weight loss and overall health.

Ron Morelli, Season 7

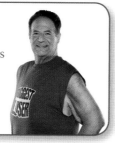

I pack a big tub of salad greens and fresh cut veggies sprinkled with balsamic vinegar to snack on throughout the day.

For starters, it helps keep your blood sugar levels balanced and stable throughout the day, preventing the peaks and crashes that can send you straight to the cookie jar. Fiber also promotes healthy cholesterol levels and decreases your risk of certain cancers. And when it comes to eating fewer calories and losing weight, fiber definitely helps you feel fuller longer.

During those first few days on campus, contestants are always shocked to learn how much food they can eat when they're eating the *right kinds* of foods. "It's blowing me away," said Season 8 contestant Danny Cahill after just 4 days of eating on the ranch. "I can't believe the volume of food I'm eating now, but with fewer calories. I was eating less food before, but way more calories."

Fresh vegetables and fruits are converted into energy much more efficiently than their processed

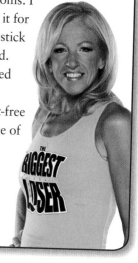

Helen Phillips, Season 7 Winner

I love portobello mushrooms. I take a big cap and steam it for about 5 minutes in a nonstick pan with a tight-fitting lid. Then I heap it with sautéed peppers and onions and sprinkle it with a little fat-free mozzarella. Throw a piece of salmon or some orange roughy on the grill and you've got a meal! My family asks me to cook this for them all the time.

versions—such as potato chips or fruit snacks sweetened with fruit juice. And fresh produce is higher in fiber, which not only helps you feel satis-

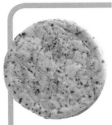

SWAP PIZZA CRUST FOR MUSHROOM CAPS.

Make a mini-pizza that satisfies your craving while cutting carbs and slashing calories. An average portobello mushroom has only 27 calories. Mushrooms have meaty texture and rich flavor, and they're loaded with antioxidants and other nutrients. Top a grilled portobello cap with tomato sauce and low-fat cheese, and you have a no-guilt pizza treat.

fied but also reduces the number of calories your body absorbs after a meal. Fresh fruits and veggies are also much lower in calories than processed foods, because they don't contain added sugar and fat. There's no mystery to a whole food—there is only one ingredient! As *Biggest Loser* trainer Bob Harper always says, "If it grows out of the ground or on a tree, chances are it's good for you!"

The Biggest Loser Plan

The Biggest Loser nutrition pyramid is made up of fruits and vegetables at its base, protein foods on the second tier, and whole grains on the third tier. The small section at the top gives you a 200-calorie budget for any food *not* included on the lower three tiers.

When you follow *The Biggest Loser* eating plan, you should eat a daily minimum of: four servings of fruits and vegetables; three servings of healthy protein; and two servings of whole grains.

Vegetables

Serving size: 1 cup or 8 ounces

Choose these to lose: Artichokes, asparagus, bamboo shoots, beans (green, yellow), beet greens,

THE 4-3-2-1 *BIGGEST LOSER* PYRAMID

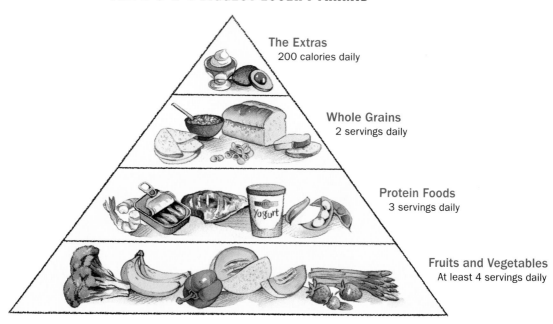

The Extras
200 calories daily

Whole Grains
2 servings daily

Protein Foods
3 servings daily

Fruits and Vegetables
At least 4 servings daily

beets, bell peppers, broccoli, brussels sprouts, cabbage, carrots, cauliflower, celery, collard greens, cucumbers, eggplant, kale, kohlrabi, leeks, lettuce (all varieties), mushrooms, mustard greens, okra, onions, palm hearts, parsley, peas, peppers (all varieties), pumpkin, radishes, shallots, spinach, sprouts, summer squash, sweet potatoes, Swiss chard, tomatillos, tomatoes, turnip greens, turnips, water chestnuts, watercress, winter squash, yams, and zucchini.

grapefruit, grapes, guava, kiwifruit, mango, melon (all varieties), nectarine, orange, papaya, peach, pear, persimmon, pineapple, plantain, plum, pomegranate, raspberries, rhubarb, strawberries, tangerine, and watermelon.

Fruit

Serving size: 1 cup, 1 medium piece, or 8 ounces

Choose these to lose: Apple, apricot, banana, blackberries, blueberries, cherries, cranberries,

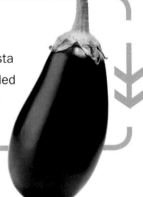

$ BUDGET TIP $
Rudy Pauls, Season 8

To save on groceries, my wife and I planted a large vegetable garden before I left for the ranch. I also plan to pack most of my meals instead of eating out.

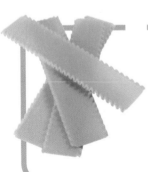 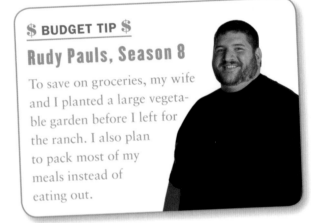

SWAP LASAGNA NOODLES FOR VEGGIES.

Try making a healthier, lower-carb lasagna by replacing the pasta in your favorite lasagna recipe with thin slices of grilled or broiled zucchini or eggplant. Better yet, try the Veggie Lasagna recipe on page 63.

Pyramid Pointers

You can eat more than four servings a day of most fruits and vegetables if you wish. The majority of your daily servings, however, should come from vegetables. At the base of our pyramid, fruits and vegetables supply most of your daily nutrients in the form of vitamins, minerals, and fiber, though they contain relatively low numbers of calories. In other words, you get the most nutritional bang for your calorie buck from fruits and vegetables. The exception to this would be the starchier vegetables, such as pumpkin, winter squash, sweet potatoes, and yams. These veggies are higher in calories and carbs, so you want to limit your intake to a few servings a week.

Fresh produce should be your first choice, but if it isn't available or is too expensive, opt for frozen or canned versions of your favorite fruits and vegetables. Just make sure there's no added salt or sugar. When it comes to dried fruit, though, be careful. When fruit is dried, it is dehydrated, meaning that all the water has been removed. So the calories in dried fruit are more concentrated. Dried fruits aren't as filling as raw fruits per serving size, but they are still a great option for portable, nonperishable snacks. When fresh fruit isn't available, dried fruits are great to sprinkle on yogurt or oatmeal or add to trail mix.

Here are some easy tips to help you meet your daily fruit and veggie requirement:

Ali Vincent, Season 5 Winner

I'm from Arizona—I love spicy foods! So salsa has turned into one of my favorite condiments. I use it all the time to kick up flavors, like adding some to a plate of sautéed veggies and chicken.

- Eat a vegetable salad most days of the week.
- Keep a container of sliced or chopped vegetables, such as broccoli, carrots, or red or green bell peppers, in your refrigerator for easy snacking.
- Choose whole fruits rather than fruit juices. Fruit juice contains no fiber and therefore does little to help you control your appetite or make you feel full.
- Try a new fruit or vegetable every week to build some variety into your diet. Choose fruits and vegetables from the six color groups: red, orange, yellow, light green, dark green, and purple. This is a great way to make sure you're getting a variety of nutrients in your diet.

- Try to eat at least one raw fruit and one raw vegetable each day.
- Mix up a fruit smoothie containing fresh or frozen fruit as a preworkout snack.

Good Food for Good Health
The Power of Antioxidants

You've probably heard a lot about antioxidants in the news lately. But what are they, and why do you need them?

Antioxidants are vitamin-like compounds that help protect your body from inflammation, diabetes, heart disease, various types of cancer, and other serious health problems. Antioxidants are found in fresh vegetables, fruits, and whole grains. Some of the most important antioxidants are vitamin A, which can be found in broccoli, cantaloupe, carrots, collard greens, potatoes, squash, and tomatoes; vitamin C, which is abundant in citrus fruit, cranberries, green peppers, leafy green

SWAP WHITE PASTA FOR SPAGHETTI SQUASH.

Spaghetti squash has been a ranch favorite since Season 2, when Suzy Hoover invented Spaghetti Squash Marinara. Season 5 winner Ali Vincent loves it, too! Not only does a cup of cooked spaghetti squash have a mere 40 calories, plus 2 grams of fiber and loads of vitamins, but it's also satisfying and flavorful. Try the Spaghetti Squash with Avocado Pesto recipe on page 68.

vegetables, and strawberries; and vitamin E, also found in leafy green vegetables, as well as in nuts, seeds, and whole grains. Another essential antioxidant is selenium, which is abundant in chicken, eggs, fish, garlic, and grains.

Different vitamins are used by our bodies in different ways. Some vitamins, such as vitamins B and C, are water soluble, which means that they stay in our bloodstream for only 4 to 6 hours. It's important to eat foods that contain these vitamins every day. Other vitamins, such as A, D, E, and K, are fat soluble, which means that they're stored in our bodies a little longer. They ensure that we stay healthy even on days when we aren't able to eat all our veggies.

Matt Kamont, Season 1

Use the cap from a salad dressing bottle to measure your salad dressing. It's usually equal to 1 tablespoon.

Aim for Vitamin A

Your body is designed to shield you from the health threats of the outside world. Therefore, your sinuses, lungs, mouth, and digestive system have a lining that makes it hard for germs to penetrate your system. One of vitamin A's most important jobs is keeping this barrier strong. When your diet is deficient in vitamin A, you can develop gaps in this barrier, allowing germs to slip through.

The best sources of vitamin A are colorful fruits and vegetables. Look for darkly colored fruits and vegetables such as cantaloupe, carrots, spinach, and sweet potatoes.

FOOD	SERVING SIZE	VITAMIN A CONTENT (INTERNATIONAL UNITS)
Spinach, cooked	½ cup	11,458
Kale, cooked	½ cup	9,558
Carrot, raw	7½ inch	8,666
Cantaloupe, cubed	1 cup	5,411
Spinach, raw	1 cup	2,813
Papaya, cubed	½ cup	766
Mango, sliced	½ cup	631
Peach	1 medium	319
Red bell pepper, raw	1 ring, 3 inches in diameter, ¼ inch thick	313

See That You Get Enough C

Health experts have long known that vitamin C plays a crucial role in helping our immune systems stay strong—that's why you've always been told to eat an orange when you feel a cold coming on.

Vitamin C is also a powerful antioxidant. The fresh fruits and vegetables in the table below are all great sources of vitamin C.

FOOD	SERVING SIZE	VITAMIN C CONTENT (MILLIGRAMS)
Red bell pepper	½ cup	95
Orange	1 medium	60
Broccoli, cooked	½ cup	60
Strawberries	½ cup	50
Papaya	½ medium	48
Green bell pepper	½ cup	45
Grapefruit, white	Half	40
Cantaloupe	½ cup	35
Mango	1 medium	30
Tangerine	1 medium	25
Cabbage greens, frozen, boiled	½ cup	25
Spinach, raw	1 cup	15

Eat Your E

When you don't have an adequate amount of the powerful antioxidant vitamin E, your immune system can become weak, making you more susceptible to illness. Lack of vitamin E can also cause inflammation. Aim to get your daily vitamin E from the foods in the table below.

FOOD	SERVING SIZE	VITAMIN E (ALPHA-TOCOPHEROL) CONTENT (MILLIGRAMS)
Almonds, dry roasted	1 tablespoon	1.8
Spinach, cooked	½ cup	1.6
Sunflower seed kernels, dry roasted	1 tablespoon	1.5
Broccoli, cooked	½ cup	1.2
Hazelnuts, dry roasted	1 tablespoon	1.1
Kiwifruit, without skin	1 medium	1.1
Mango, peeled, seeded, and sliced	½ cup	0.9
Spinach, raw	1 cup	0.6
Peanuts, dry roasted	1 tablespoon	0.6

Select Selenium

Selenium is also an important player in preventing the development of chronic diseases such as cancer and heart disease. Selenium may also help regulate thyroid function. You'll find it in the following foods.

FOOD	SERVING SIZE	SELENIUM CONTENT (MICROGRAMS)
Brazil nut, dried	1 large	91
Cod, cooked	3 ounces	32
Turkey, light meat, roasted	3½ ounces	32
Chicken breast, skinless, roasted	3½ ounces	20
Egg, whole	1 medium	14
Cottage cheese, fat free	½ cup	12
Rice, brown, long-grain, cooked	½ cup	10
Garlic, chopped	2 tablespoons	2.5

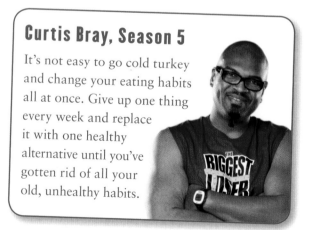

Curtis Bray, Season 5

It's not easy to go cold turkey and change your eating habits all at once. Give up one thing every week and replace it with one healthy alternative until you've gotten rid of all your old, unhealthy habits.

Jicama

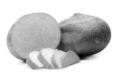

Jicama is one of my favorite ingredients to introduce to the contestants because so many of them have never tasted it before—but once they do, they all love it! It's a welcome addition to salads, and I also love to cut it in thin chips or thick strips for a crunchy snack. It's delicious with a squeeze of fresh lime and a sprinkle of chili powder. Whole jicama keeps well in the fridge for about 3 weeks; once cut, it lasts about 1 week. One cup has 45 calories and provides 40 percent of your recommended daily vitamin C.

Shallots

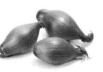

It's easy for chefs to forget that not everyone knows the value of these fabulous little bulbs. I was reminded recently when Season 7 contestant Cathy Skell told me she had never tried a recipe containing shallots because she didn't know how to use them. A small amount of chopped shallots adds loads of flavor to just about anything—from a vegetable stir-fry to a whole grain dish or a scrumptious omelet. Shallots are usually found near the onions in the produce department and should be stored the same way: in a cool area for a few weeks.

Chard

Green or red chard is a flavorful leafy green that's easy to find, easy to prepare, and easy on the pocketbook. Though it's delicious on its own, the leaves can be torn or shredded and stirred into a soup or a grain dish for extra color, flavor, and texture. Chard is loaded with vitamins: One cup of cooked chard delivers 210 percent of your recommended daily vitamin A, 50 percent of your vitamin C, 4 grams of fiber, and only 35 calories.

Eggplant

An eggplant is 95 percent water, which means it's very low in calories. A $1\frac{1}{2}$-pound eggplant yields about 5 cups of diced (uncooked) eggplant with just over 100 calories. Eggplants have a dimple at the blossom end that can be round or oval in shape. An oval dimple is usually shallower and often indicative of fewer seeds and a meatier, more desirable eggplant. When shopping for eggplant, look for smooth skin that yields slightly to pressure but bounces back. A fresh eggplant should seem heavy for its size. It's best to cook an eggplant right away. Its neutral flavor profile means that eggplant combines well with other vegetables and seasonings.

SWAP FRUIT FOR TOMATO SALSA.

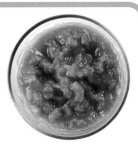

This swap is a favorite at the ranch. Instead of pairing cottage cheese with something sweet, add ½ cup of salsa to ½ cup of cottage cheese. A half cup of salsa satisfies one of your daily vegetable servings and contains only 21 calories. Salsa is also a great replacement for sour cream on your quesadilla or burrito—a savings of more than 200 calories per ½ cup.

SWAP POTATO CHIPS FOR JICAMA CHIPS.

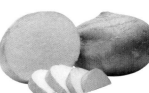

Also known as the Mexican potato, jicama is a sweet edible root that makes a delicious impostor for your favorite dip. One cup of raw jicama slices contains 45 calories, 6 grams of fiber, and nearly 40 percent of your daily vitamin C!

SWAP POTATOES FOR OTHER ROOT VEGETABLES.

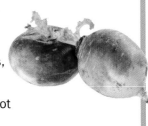

Like pasta, potatoes are a downfall for many people. Try replacing potatoes with other root vegetables (turnips, parsnips, rutabagas) and roasting them with fresh herbs, olive oil, and a sprinkle of salt. Check out the recipe for Rosemary-Roasted Root Vegetables on page 64.

SWAP CELERY AND CARROTS FOR BELL PEPPERS.

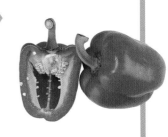

The next time you pack veggie sticks for a snack, pass on the celery or carrots and try bell pepper slices instead. They're loaded with antioxidants and are a rich source of vitamin C. One cup of bell pepper slices has only 20 calories and packs 120 percent of your daily supply of vitamin C.

FRESH TOMATO SALAD WITH LEMON AND CILANTRO

This simple salad is especially refreshing and delicious in the summer, when tomatoes are in season and at the height of their flavor.

2 large ripe tomatoes, diced (see note)

1 medium stalk celery, halved lengthwise and thinly sliced

½ yellow bell pepper, finely chopped

¼ cup chopped fresh cilantro

¼ cup chopped fresh Italian parsley

2 tablespoons lemon peel

1 tablespoon finely chopped fresh ginger

1 tablespoon balsamic vinegar

¾ teaspoon ground cumin

In a mixing bowl, combine the tomatoes, celery, bell pepper, cilantro, parsley, lemon peel, ginger, vinegar, and cumin. Serve immediately or refrigerate for a few hours to allow the flavors to blend.

Note: If fresh tomatoes aren't available, use 2 cups canned diced fire-roasted tomatoes.

Makes 4 servings

Per serving: 21 calories, 1 g protein, 5 g carbohydrates, 0 g fat (0 g saturated), 0 mg cholesterol, 2 g fiber, 21 mg sodium

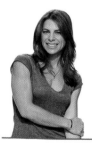

Trainer Tip: JILLIAN MICHAELS

Combining the right foods can help you improve your overall health. For example, at breakfast have some cantaloupe along with your eggs. Research shows that combining protein, carbs, and fat can increase fullness and will help you sustain your energy level.

ROSEMARY-ROASTED ROOT VEGETABLES

The secret to perfect roasting is a hot oven and a large enough pan to eliminate crowding. This ensures a crispy exterior and even browning. You can change the proportions of the vegetables if you like; just be sure they're cut the same size for uniform baking. Butternut squash or sweet potatoes work well, too.

16 ounces any combination of parsnips, rutabagas, or turnips, peeled and cut in 1" pieces

2 teaspoons olive oil

1 teaspoon chopped fresh rosemary

1 teaspoon chopped fresh thyme

½ teaspoon ground mustard

¼ teaspoon salt

¼ teaspoon ground black pepper

Preheat the oven to 400°F. Place the parsnips, rutabagas, and turnips on a 15" × 10" baking sheet. Drizzle with the oil and sprinkle with the rosemary, thyme, mustard, and salt. Toss well and distribute evenly over the pan. Roast, stirring or shaking the vegetables every 15 minutes, until they're tender and evenly browned, or about 45 minutes. Sprinkle with black pepper; taste and adjust the seasonings. Serve hot or at room temperature.

Makes 4 servings

Per serving: 70 calories, 1 g protein, 13 g carbohydrates, 2 g fat (0 g saturated), 0 mg cholesterol, 3 g fiber, 180 mg sodium

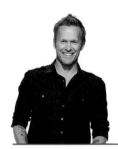

Trainer Tip: BOB HARPER

Here's a trick when trying to cut calories: Eat the low-calorie items in any meal first, such as salad, veggies, and soup. Eat the meats and starches last. By the time you get to them, you'll be full enough to eat smaller portions of the higher-fat, higher-calorie items.

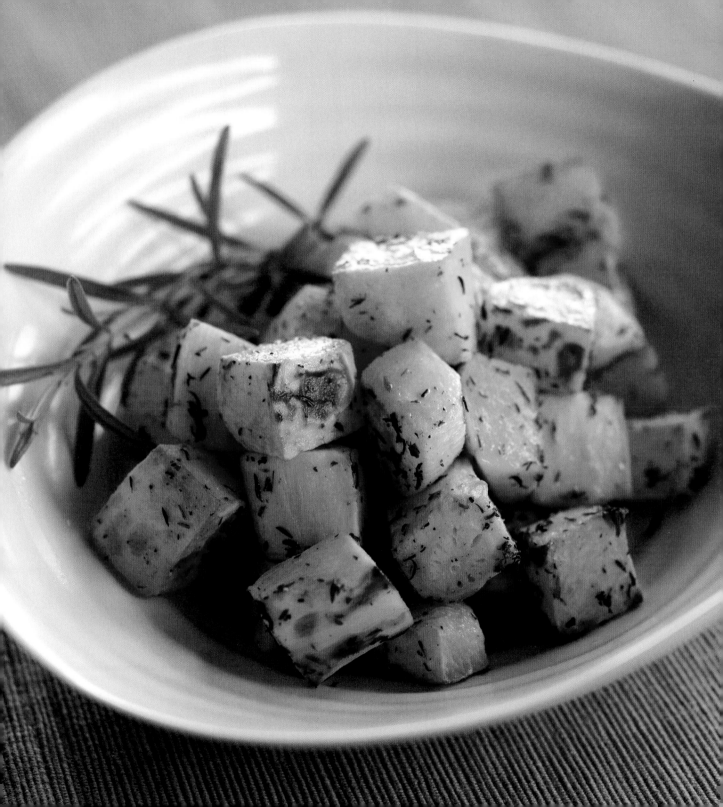

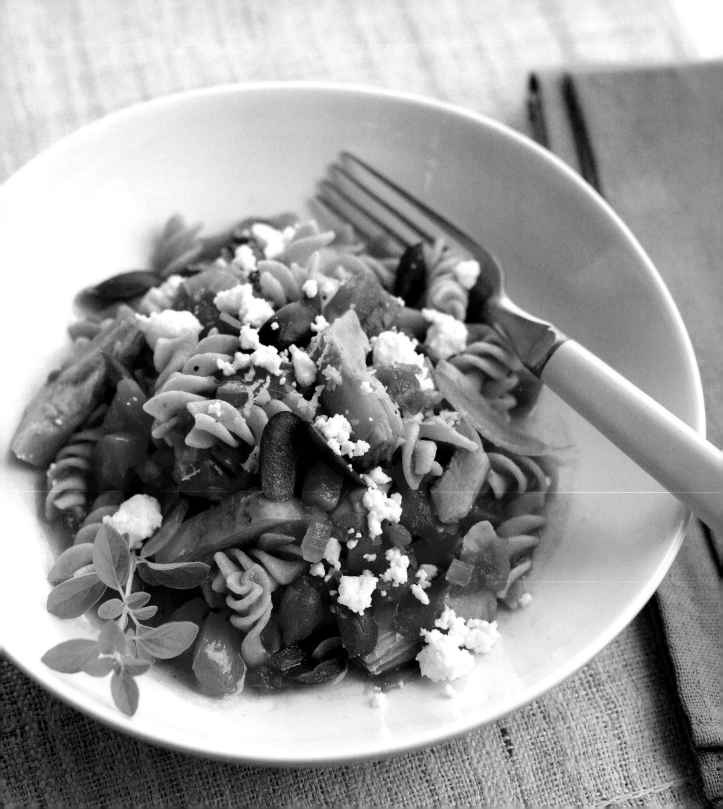

GREEK-STYLE PASTA WITH FIRE-ROASTED TOMATO SAUCE AND CRUMBLED FETA CHEESE

This dish is upside down—it's heavy on the sauce! You'll still enjoy the same portion of food, but you'll take in many fewer calories when you kick up the sauce and veggies and dial down the pasta. This recipe is great hot or cold as a side dish. Add grilled chicken or shrimp and you have a meal!

6 ounces whole grain penne or fusilli (I use Healthy Harvest brand)

2 teaspoons olive oil

1 medium onion, chopped

1 tablespoon minced garlic

1 red bell pepper, finely chopped

3 cups (about 28 ounces) fire-roasted tomatoes

1 (8-ounce) package frozen artichoke hearts, thawed and halved lengthwise

¼ cup crumbled low-fat feta cheese

8 kalamata or other black olives, sliced

1 tablespoon fresh lemon peel

Fresh Italian parsley or oregano (optional)

Prepare the pasta al dente according to package directions. Drain and set aside.

In a large nonstick skillet, heat the oil over medium-high heat. Add the onion and cook for about 5 minutes, or until soft and just starting to brown. Add the garlic and simmer for 1 minute longer, but do not allow the garlic to brown. Add the bell pepper and cook just until softened.

Add the tomatoes and simmer for about 4 minutes. Gently add the artichokes and cook for 1 minute longer, or until just heated through.

Pour the sauce into a large mixing bowl and add the cooked pasta. Toss lightly and transfer to a serving bowl. Top with the cheese, olives, and lemon peel.

Divide between serving bowls and garnish with parsley or oregano if desired. Serve hot or at room temperature.

Makes 8 (about 1-cup) side dish servings or 4 main course servings

Per serving: 140 calories, 7 g protein, 27 g carbohydrates, 3 g fat (less than 1 g saturated), 5 mg cholesterol, 6 g fiber, 410 mg sodium

SPAGHETTI SQUASH WITH AVOCADO PESTO

This flavorful squash can always be found in the kitchen at the ranch as a creative replacement for white pasta. Add grilled chicken and a tomato salad and you have a meal. The avocado pesto is also delicious as a sandwich condiment or drizzled over sliced tomatoes.

1 medium spaghetti squash (1½–2 pounds), washed, halved lengthwise, and seeded

½ ripe avocado, pitted and diced

¼ cup fresh basil leaves or Italian parsley

1 tablespoon chopped chives

2 tablespoons grated Parmesan cheese

1 teaspoon minced garlic

½ teaspoon salt

¼ teaspoon ground black pepper

⅓ cup hot water

2 tablespoons chopped fresh basil or parsley (optional)

Preheat the oven to 375°F. Lightly coat a baking sheet with olive oil cooking spray.

Pierce the outside of each half of the squash a few times with a fork. Place the squash cut side down on the baking sheet and bake for about 45 minutes, or until very tender when tested with a fork. Cool slightly.

Meanwhile, place the avocado, basil or parsley, chives, Parmesan, garlic, salt, black pepper, and hot water in a blender and process until smooth, turning the blender off and on occasionally and adding a tablespoon or two of additional hot water if needed. There will be between ½ and ¾ cup of pesto.

When the squash has cooled, use a fork to rake the spaghetti-like threads of squash into a serving bowl. Discard the skin. There will be about 3 cups of spaghetti squash. Drizzle the pesto over the squash and garnish with fresh basil or parsley if desired.

Makes 6 servings

Per serving: 60 calories, 2 g protein, 9 g carbohydrates, 3 g fat (0 g saturated), 0 mg cholesterol, 3 g fiber, 230 mg sodium

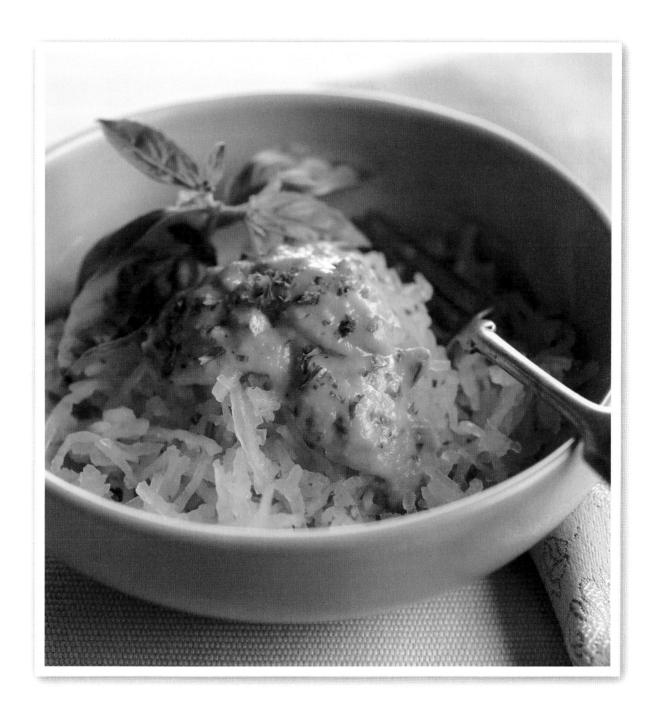

ROASTED TAMALE CHILI

The smoky flavors of fire-roasted tomatoes and (optional) addition of chipotle chile peppers create a rich and satisfying vegetarian chili. Kidney beans, pinto beans, or navy beans can be substituted for the black beans. Leftovers freeze well, so you can make a big batch on the weekend and defrost single servings during the week.

- 1 tablespoon olive oil
- 1 large yellow onion, diced
- 1 green bell pepper, seeded and diced
- 1 tablespoon chopped garlic
- ⅓ cup chopped sun-dried tomatoes
- 3 cups (28 ounces) fire-roasted crushed tomatoes
- 1 (15-ounce) can (1½ cups) cooked black beans, rinsed and drained
- 2 teaspoons chili powder
- 1 tablespoon chopped fresh oregano or 1 teaspoon dried
- 1 teaspoon ground cumin
- 1 teaspoon chopped chipotle chile peppers (optional; see note)
- Salt, to taste
- 3 cups fat-free, reduced-sodium chicken broth or vegetable broth
- ⅓ cup masa harina (stone-ground cornmeal, finely ground)
- ¼ cup chopped fresh cilantro
- ¼ cup chopped chives or scallions

Heat the oil in a large saucepan. Add the onion and bell pepper and cook for 6 to 8 minutes, or until tender. Add the garlic and cook for 1 minute longer, but don't allow the garlic to brown. Stir in the sun-dried tomatoes, roasted tomatoes, beans, chili powder, oregano, cumin, chile peppers (if desired), salt, and 1 cup of the broth. Bring to a simmer and cook uncovered over low heat, stirring occasionally, for about 5 minutes. Keep hot.

Meanwhile, in a 1-quart saucepan, bring the remaining 2 cups of broth to a boil. Reduce the heat to low and whisk in the masa harina. Cook gently for about 4 minutes, or until the mixture has thickened slightly. Remove from the heat and carefully pour the masa broth into the bean mixture. Add the cilantro and stir well. Ladle the chili into bowls and garnish with chives or scallions.

Makes 8 (about 1-cup) servings (about 2 quarts)

Note: Chipotle chile peppers, canned in a spicy sauce called adobo, are available at Latin American markets, specialty foods stores, and some supermarkets. Leftover canned chile peppers can be transferred to a glass jar and stored in the refrigerator. Dried chipotle peppers can be rehydrated and used instead of the canned ones.

Per serving: 120 calories, 5 g protein, 21 g carbohydrates, 2 g fat (0 g saturated), 0 mg cholesterol, 5 g fiber, 450 mg sodium

Mushrooms

Mushrooms are so underrated! Loaded with nutrients, they're also very high in water (which makes them filling) and low in calories. A great addition to salads and stir-fries, they're also delicious when stuffed and baked. Large mushrooms are excellent when grilled and make a great replacement for meat in a veggie burger. When buying fresh mushrooms, make sure they are firm. Store them, wrapped loosely in plastic, in the refrigerator.

SWAP BREAD FOR LETTUCE.

Give your sandwich a protein makeover by tossing those white buns and wrapping your burger or sandwich fixings in a leaf or two of romaine. When you do have a serious bread craving, be sure to choose whole grain bread.

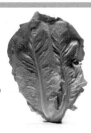

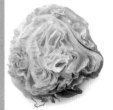

SWAP ICEBERG FOR SPINACH.

Instead of the usual iceberg lettuce, try using spinach or romaine in your salads and sandwiches. These darker greens contain more nutrients and add a different flavor and texture to your salad.

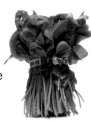

SWAP MEAT FOR VEGETABLES.

Forget the meat in your next batch of chili and kick up the flavor with roasted bell peppers, a variety of beans, and some extra herbs and spices. Try black, pinto, white, or navy beans, and sprinkle in some cumin or fresh cilantro. Or try the Roasted Tamale Chili recipe on the opposite page.

it to work, firing it up and tossing on chicken, fish, lean cuts of meat, and veggies. (One of trainer Bob Harper's tricks is to grill brussels sprouts, which he says makes them taste just like potatoes.) When the weather's not conducive to grilling, contestants make use of big grill pans on the stove for grilling or sautéing meat family-style.

Rebecca Meyer, Season 8

I'm from the Midwest, so I'm used to cooking chicken-fried steak with mashed potatoes and green bean casserole. At the ranch I've learned to make stuffed chicken breasts with low-fat cheese, spinach, and garlic. I eat one with broccoli and brown rice for a new healthy meal.

"I love grilling," Bob says. "I love thinking about all the excess fat just dripping off the meat."

It may look as if the contestants at the ranch are spoiled, but at the end of the day, when they're exhausted from tough workouts and utterly fatigued, they still have to prepare their own healthy dinners! Danny Cahill of Season 8 learned early on the importance of planning ahead. "I have dinner in the fridge," he said one afternoon while working out. "I'm going to microwave it when I get back and have a nice meal that's three or four hundred calories and that's going to fill me up. Before, if I wanted something quick and easy, I'd stop at a drive-thru!"

In this chapter, you'll learn how to swap healthy proteins for the not-so-healthy ones you may be used to. You'll find much more nutritious—and tasty—options for your meals than a greasy burger on the run!

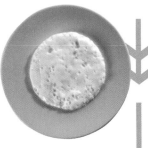

SWAP EGG YOLKS FOR WHITES.

Cutting back on egg yolks slashes cholesterol and cuts calories by 75 percent. That's because the yolk is nearly all fat (and the white is nearly pure protein). To make a gradual change, use one whole egg mixed with three whites in your next omelet or scramble. Compared with three whole eggs, you'll save 100 calories and 9 grams of fat, and increase the protein by 25 percent.

SWAP PEAS FOR EDAMAME.

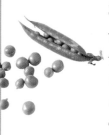

The similar appearance of these two pale green pods belies the fact that they're very different nutritionally *and* flavor-wise. Edamame are loaded with heart-healthy fats and contain twice as much protein as peas do. So while edamame have a few more calories, you can eat less of them and feel fuller. Try the Smoky "Pea" Soup recipe on page 86.

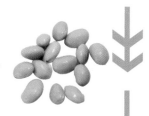

Protein Primer

The second tier of *The Biggest Loser* food pyramid (see page 53) is all about protein. Not only is protein a valuable source of energy, but it also helps with hunger control and promotes weight loss and fat burning.

Protein Facts

Protein is a macronutrient found in meat, fish, eggs, poultry, and dairy products, and in smaller amounts in beans, nuts, and whole grains. Protein is required to build and repair muscle, skin, hair, blood vessels, and other bodily tissues. Generally speaking, anything above 9 grams of protein per serving means the food is a high-protein food.

Lean proteins contain valuable nutrients that can help you achieve a healthy weight, and they have the added benefit of slowing the aging process. Proteins deliver calcium, iron, selenium, and zinc, which are essential for building strong bones, fighting cancer, and protecting your immune system. Protein is also required for making and preserving muscle and for repairing tissue, so it's especially important to get your daily requirement when you're hitting the gym hard.

Try to eat a little bit of protein within 30 minutes after a workout to help your muscles repair quickly. You could have a turkey sandwich or some low-fat

Nutritionist Tip

Consider purchasing free-range or grass-fed meat or poultry. These foods contain more healthy fats and less saturated fat than conventionally raised meats and are free of antibiotics and growth hormones.

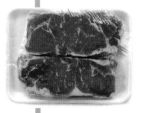

SWAP MEAT FOR BEANS OR TOFU IN YOUR NEXT CURRY.

Beans and other legumes are not only very inexpensive; they also have antiaging properties! They're excellent sources of folic acid, calcium, iron, potassium, zinc, and antioxidants, and they provide steady energy because of their abundance of complex carbs, fiber, and protein. Try the Vegetarian Curry Stew recipe on page 91.

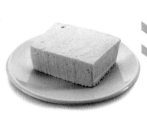

yogurt or cottage cheese, or nibble on steamed edamame. Half a cup of these pale green soybeans contains a whopping 14 grams of protein! Include protein with each meal and each snack so your body can benefit all day long. When you haven't eaten enough protein, you might find yourself running low on energy or suffering from muscle fatigue at the end of a demanding day.

In addition to helping build muscle, protein, like fiber, also promotes the feeling of satiety, or fullness, thus curbing your appetite and keeping you from consuming extra calories. When combined with a carbohydrate (such as a piece of fruit), protein helps slow the release of blood sugar, minimizing unhealthy spikes and sustaining our energy for longer periods of time.

Choose a variety of proteins each day. For example, at breakfast, you might have a cup of yogurt; at

lunch, a cup of kidney beans as part of a vegetarian chili; for a snack, ½ cup of cottage cheese; and for dinner, 4 ounces of grilled salmon.

30 Percent Protein

On *The Biggest Loser* eating plan, approximately 30 percent of your daily calorie intake comes from lean

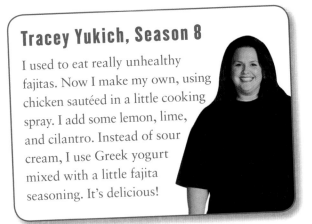

Tracey Yukich, Season 8

I used to eat really unhealthy fajitas. Now I make my own, using chicken sautéed in a little cooking spray. I add some lemon, lime, and cilantro. Instead of sour cream, I use Greek yogurt mixed with a little fajita seasoning. It's delicious!

protein. There are three main kinds of protein: lean animal protein, low-fat or fat-free dairy protein, and vegetarian protein. Choose a variety of proteins each day in order to meet your calorie goal.

To figure out how many grams of protein you need each day, follow this formula, which uses a 1,500-calorie budget as an example.

$$1,500 \times 0.30 = 450 \text{ calories from protein}$$

Then convert the calories to grams.

$$450 \div 4 \text{ calories per gram} = 112.5 \text{ grams of}$$
protein required each day, which we'll round down to 112

Now break it down to grams of protein per meal and snack.

Breakfast	28 grams
Snack 1	14 grams
Lunch	28 grams
Snack 2	14 grams
Dinner	28 grams

Animal Protein

Serving size: *1 cup or 8 ounces*

Meat

Choose lean cuts of beef and pork, such as bottom round, eye of round, flank steak, sirloin tip, top round, top sirloin, and pork tenderloin. USDA Choice or USDA Select grades of beef usually have lower fat content. Avoid meat that is heavily marbled with fat and remove any visible fat. Try to find ground meat that's at least 95 percent lean. Limit red meat servings to two a week, since red meat tends to be higher in saturated fat than other animal protein. And avoid processed meats, such as

SWAP TRADITIONAL YOGURT FOR GREEK-STYLE YOGURT.

Greek-style fat-free yogurt contains the same number of calories as regular fat-free yogurt (approximately 100 per cup) but has twice the protein and half the carbs. Its velvety texture makes a great base for dips, too. Try using it in the French Onion Dip recipe on page 88.

SWAP TUNA FOR SALMON.

The next time you want to mix up some tuna salad, opt for a can of water-packed salmon instead. The calories and protein are the same as in tuna, but salmon is higher in heart-healthy omega-3 fats, and it contains 10 times more calcium than tuna.

bologna, hot dogs, and sausage; they're generally high in fat, sodium, and calories. They may also contain sodium nitrites, which can form carcinogenic (potentially cancer-causing) compounds.

Poultry

Skinless white meat from the breast of a chicken or turkey is the best option. When choosing ground chicken or turkey, ask for the white meat. And before cooking poultry, always remove the skin. This greatly reduces the fat and calorie content.

Seafood

Sefood is an excellent source of protein, omega-3 fatty acids, vitamin E, and selenium. When you're buying seafood, go for options that are rich in omega-3 fatty acids, such as herring, mackerel, salmon, sardines (water packed), trout, and tuna. Cold-water fish contain more heart-healthy fats—but be careful with serving sizes, as these types of fish also have more calories.

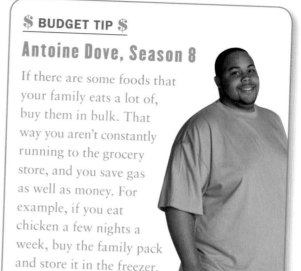

$ BUDGET TIP $

Antoine Dove, Season 8

If there are some foods that your family eats a lot of, buy them in bulk. That way you aren't constantly running to the grocery store, and you save gas as well as money. For example, if you eat chicken a few nights a week, buy the family pack and store it in the freezer.

Choose these to lose: Any type of beef, pork, or veal labeled as 95 percent lean; fish and seafood, including herring, mackerel, salmon, sardines (water packed), trout, and tuna; white meat chicken; and white meat turkey.

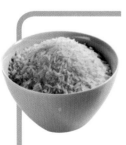

SWAP RICE FOR LENTILS.

Next time you're whipping up your favorite rice or couscous dish, kick up the protein and fiber levels by stirring in lentils instead. A half cup of cooked lentils has a whopping 10 grams of protein.

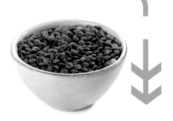

LEAN ANIMAL PROTEIN NUTRIENTS

PROTEIN SOURCE (3 OUNCES RAW)	CALORIES	PROTEIN (GRAMS)	FAT (GRAMS)
Ground turkey breast, 1% fat	91	20	1
Eye of round, lean	103	19	3
Bottom round, lean	114	18	4
Pork tenderloin, lean	112	18	4
Skinless chicken breast	102	18	2.5
Top round, lean	100	18	3
Tri tip, lean	107	18	3
Ground turkey breast, 7% fat	122	17	6
Top sirloin, lean	101	17	3

Dairy

Serving size: *1 cup or 8 ounces*

Dairy products are prime sources of protein as well as calcium, a vital nutrient for your body's bones and muscles, including the heart. As calcium is found in the fat-free part of milk, choosing lower-fat dairy foods will not detract from your calcium intake. Low-fat yogurts, however, aren't always healthier than the full-fat options, because the fat is often replaced with extra sugar and thickeners to improve the flavor and texture. Adults need 1,000 milligrams of bone-building calcium daily. One cup of plain, low-fat yogurt contains about 425 milligrams of calcium.

Choose these to lose: Fat-free (skim) milk, low-fat (1%) milk, buttermilk, plain fat-free or low-fat Greek-style yogurt, fat-free or low-fat yogurt with fruit (no sugar added), fat-free or low-fat cottage cheese, and fat-free or low-fat ricotta cheese. Light soymilks and soy yogurts can also be used.

SWAP YOUR CHEESE.

Cheese is a great source of protein, calcium, and phosphorus, but it can also be a major source of calories and fat, including saturated fat, which contains cholesterol. Switching to fat-free, low-fat, or reduced-fat cheeses will deliver big savings in the calorie department.

Vegetarian Protein

Serving size: *1 cup or 8 ounces*

Excellent sources of vegetarian protein include beans, other legumes, and a variety of soy foods. Many are also loaded with fiber. Consider eating soy foods such as soy hot dogs, soy sausage, and even soy pastrami, because they contain no saturated fat. You can find them at your local natural foods store and in many grocery stores.

Some of the complex sugars that beans and legumes contain are hard to digest. To avoid intestinal discomfort, soak dry beans as directed on the package before cooking. This helps dissolve the complex sugars and minimizes unpleasant side effects. Supplemental enzymes are also available over the counter to help you digest the complex sugars. They can be taken just before your first bite of food.

Choose these to lose: Black beans, broad beans,

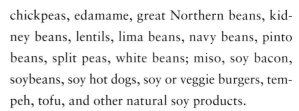

SWAP CHICKEN BREAST FOR TURKEY BREAST.

Turkey's not just for Thanksgiving anymore—this healthy protein is a great choice year round. Both of these lean meats are healthy options, but turkey is lower in calories *and* fat. Turkey is often less expensive, too. Try the Tangy Turkey Wrap recipe on page 92.

chickpeas, edamame, great Northern beans, kidney beans, lentils, lima beans, navy beans, pinto beans, split peas, white beans; miso, soy bacon, soybeans, soy hot dogs, soy or veggie burgers, tempeh, tofu, and other natural soy products.

Soy foods are good sources of protein and fiber. The chart below contains nutrient values for common soy foods.

SOY FOOD NUTRIENTS

SOY FOOD	PROTEIN (GRAMS)	FIBER (GRAMS)	CALORIES
White soybeans (½ cup)	14	4	149
Tofu, firm (4 ounces)	12	1	103
Black soybeans (½ cup)	11	7	120
Tempeh (2 ounces)	11	3	110
Roasted soy nuts (¼ cup)	8	1	106
Frozen edamame (½ cup)	6	6	100
Roasted soy butter (2 tablespoons)	6	1	80
Light soy milk (1 cup)	4	2	90

SWAP WATER OR BROTH FOR MILK.

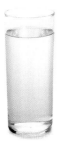

Though *The Biggest Loser* eating plan encourages you to eat, not drink, your calories, milk is an exception. That's because most of us aren't meeting our daily calcium requirement to build and maintain strong bones. The next time you make hot cereal or soup, try swapping part of the water or broth for milk. You'll get a richer flavor and a calcium boost. Try the Hi-Pro Vanilla Breakfast Grains recipe on page 92.

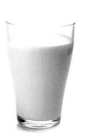

Adding Protein to Your Daily Menu

Protein sources vary widely in calories, so make sure you choose foods that fit into your calorie budget. The following guidelines will help you select the right protein-rich foods for your calorie budget.

Nutritionist Tip

You can find calcium in dairy foods, of course, but did you know that leafy green vegetables, canned wild salmon, and tofu are also great sources of calcium? If you're lactose intolerant or have a dairy allergy, there are plenty of ways to get your daily calcium.

- **Lower calorie budgets (1,050 to 1,400 calories):** Low-fat dairy will most often be your protein of choice, because it's low in calories and because the calcium in dairy foods is especially important for bone health in people with lower caloric needs. *The Biggest Loser* eating plan recommends that you get your three daily servings as follows: two servings of low-fat dairy and one serving of animal protein, vegetarian protein, or a combination of the two.

- **Midrange calorie budgets (1,401 to 1,800 calories):** *The Biggest Loser* eating plan recommends that you get your three daily servings as follows: one to two servings of low-fat dairy and one to two servings of animal protein, vegetarian protein, or a combination of the two.

- **Higher calorie budgets (1,801 to 2,100 calories):** *The Biggest Loser* eating plan recommends that you get your three daily servings as follows: one serving of low-fat dairy and two servings of animal protein.

Protein sources such as egg whites, beans, and soy foods are excellent daily protein choices for everyone, regardless of your caloric goals.

Spice It Up!

Instead of making the same old chicken breasts or ground turkey for dinner, add flavor to your healthy protein with your own Italian Seasoning Blend. This versatile blend of dried herbs works well with tomato sauce (try it with turkey meatballs or lasagna) or as a flavoring for omelets, soups, and more. Feel free to change the ratios if you favor one herb over the other. Combine 1 tablespoon dried basil, 2 teaspoons dried marjoram, 1 teaspoon dried thyme, 1 teaspoon dried oregano, and ½ teaspoon dried sage. Stir or shake to combine and store in an airtight jar or zip-top bag. Add a teaspoon (or more, to taste) to your next Italian favorite!

Antoine Dove, Season 8

On the ranch, I've been eating fruit in salads. I'll cut up strawberries and put them in the salad. The juice serves as a kind of natural dressing and sweetens it up. It's good! I'm learning how to get the most out of my calories for the day.

Fat-Free Greek-Style Yogurt

Fat-free Greek-style yogurt is strained more than other yogurts. This removes more of the watery whey and makes the yogurt thicker. Since whey is mostly carbohydrate, the strained yogurt contains less carbohydrate and consequently more protein. Its rich, creamy texture belies the fact that it contains no fat. Great as a substitute for sour cream in dips and toppings as well as a delicious dessert with berries, Greek-style yogurt can deliver as much as 20 grams of protein per serving.

Edamame

Edamame take only a few minutes to cook and are usually boiled or steamed. They are commonly found in the frozen vegetable aisle of the grocery store. An excellent source of protein and fiber, ½ cup of shelled edamame delivers 100 calories, 8 grams of protein, and 4 grams of fiber. Delicious alone as a snack, they're also a fabulous high-protein swap for sweet peas. Try the Smoky "Pea" Soup recipe on page 86.

Pork Tenderloin

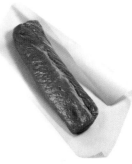

Many *Biggest Loser* contestants fear I'm going to make them give up meat forever. I love telling them about pork tenderloin, because nutritionally, it's very similar to turkey or chicken breast. Three ounces of lean pork tenderloin has 112 calories, 18 grams of protein, and 4 grams of fat. It's a great addition to a stir-fry, and it's easy to marinate and then bake or toss on the grill.

Egg Whites

The white of an egg is the purest form of protein. One large egg white has nearly 4 grams of protein and only 17 calories. When cooking or baking, you can substitute egg whites for whole eggs using the following conversions: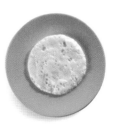
3 tablespoons egg whites = 1 whole egg;
2 tablespoons egg whites = 1 egg white; and
½ cup egg whites = 4 to 5 egg whites.

SMOKY "PEA" SOUP

Edamame are immature soybeans. They are rich in protein and fiber and have a slightly nutty flavor. They are delicious in this creamy, flavorful version of a traditional pea soup.

½ cup (about 3 slices or 2 ounces) chopped Canadian bacon

1 teaspoon olive oil

½ cup chopped yellow onion

1 teaspoon chopped garlic

1 (15½-ounce) can (2 cups) fat-free, low-sodium chicken broth

1 cup 1% milk

1 teaspoon dried sage

½ teaspoon ground cumin

½ teaspoon salt

¾ pound (about 2 cups) shelled edamame

Salt and ground black pepper

6 tablespoons plain, fat-free Greek-style yogurt

2 tablespoons chopped scallions or chives

In a small nonstick skillet, lightly brown the bacon. Set aside.

In a 3-quart nonstick saucepan, heat the oil over medium heat. Add the onion and cook for about 4 minutes, or until softened but not browned. Add the garlic and cook for about 1 minute longer, but don't allow the garlic to brown. Add the broth, milk, sage, cumin, and salt and bring to a boil. Add the edamame and reduce the heat to low. Simmer for about 3 minutes. Carefully pour the mixture into a blender and puree until smooth.

Return the puree to the saucepan and stir in the bacon. Season with salt and pepper. Pour the hot soup into 6 small bowls. Garnish with a dollop of yogurt and sprinkle with scallions or chives.

Makes 6 (¾-cup) servings

Per serving: 130 calories, 11 g protein, 12 g carbohydrates, 4 g fat (less than 1 g saturated), 5 mg cholesterol, 3 g fiber, 390 mg sodium

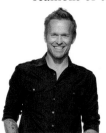

Trainer Tip: BOB HARPER

Many people are wary of soy, but they shouldn't be. This inexpensive, high-quality protein contains fiber, vitamins, and minerals. It's known to prevent cardiovascular disease, and it's easy to find at your local grocery store. Try soy milk, tofu hot dogs, or soy protein bars to keep your muscles strong and your heart healthy.

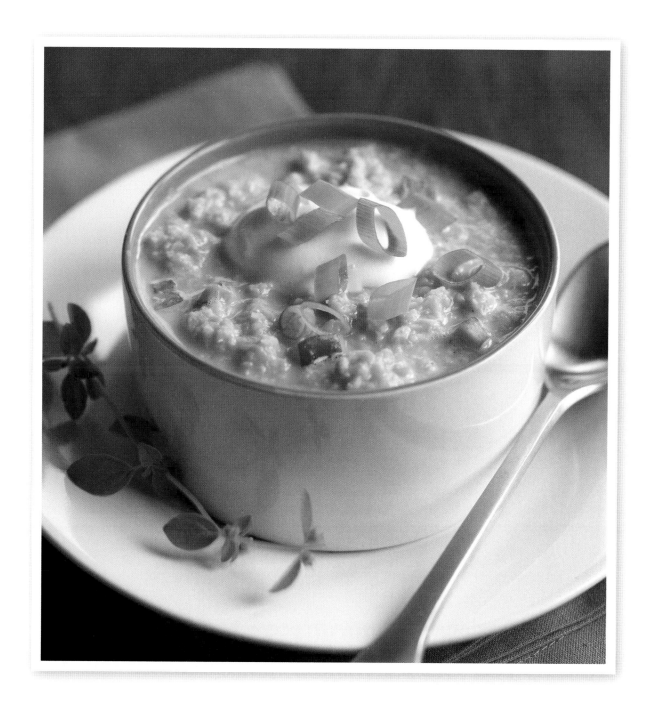

FRENCH ONION DIP

It takes a little time to simmer the onions, but the result is worth waiting for. This tastes just like "the real thing" but has a fraction of the calories and fat. Serve with jicama chips instead of potato chips and you have a double swap!

1 tablespoon olive oil

2¼ pounds yellow onions, peeled, halved vertically, and sliced horizontally into ⅛"-thick half-rounds

1 teaspoon salt

1 teaspoon onion powder

4 ounces low-fat cream cheese, at room temperature

½ cup plain, fat-free Greek-style yogurt

2 teaspoons Italian parsley, chopped

In a large skillet or Dutch oven, heat the oil over medium heat. Add the onions and salt. Stir well and cook for 2 to 3 minutes. Continue to simmer, stirring regularly, for 20 to 30 minutes, scraping up any browned bits with a wooden spoon. The onions will be light to medium golden brown (not dark brown) and caramelized. Cool the onions completely.

Place the onions in the bowl of a food processor. Pulse a few times, until they're slightly chopped. Remove half of the onions and transfer them to a mixing bowl. To the remaining onions in the food processor, add the onion powder and process until completely pureed. Add the cream cheese and yogurt and process just until smooth. Add this mixture to the chopped onions in the mixing bowl and stir well.

Taste and adjust the seasonings as desired, then chill completely. Transfer to a serving bowl. Garnish with Italian parsley leaves and serve with jicama slices or your favorite baked chips.

Makes 12 (¼-cup) servings

Per serving (¼ cup dip with ½ cup jicama slices): 80 calories, 4 g protein, 10 g carbohydrates, 3 g fat (1 g saturated), 5 mg cholesterol, 2 g fiber, 230 mg sodium

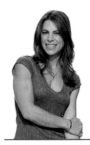

Trainer Tip: JILLIAN MICHAELS

Losing weight is not about starving yourself; it's about eating what you want with certain modifications.

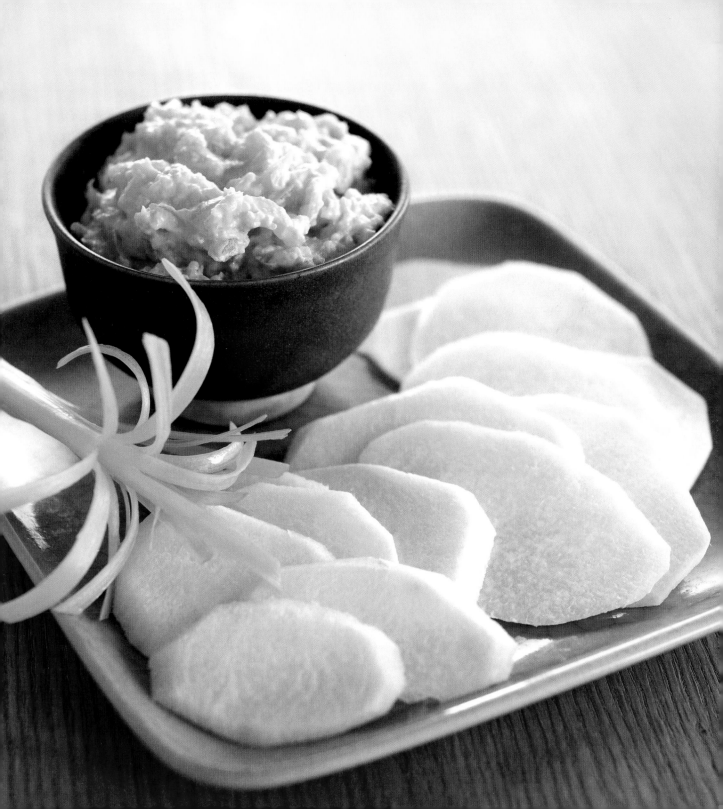

SPICY, CRUNCHY CHICKPEAS

These flavorful baked chickpeas make an excellent snack and are a great swap for oil-roasted nuts. They are also a delicious source of fiber and protein sprinkled on your favorite veggie salad.

1 (15-ounce) can chickpeas or 1½ cups cooked chickpeas, drained, rinsed, and patted dry

1 teaspoon olive oil

1 teaspoon ground coriander

½ teaspoon curry powder

½ teaspoon red chili flakes (optional)

¼ teaspoon salt

¼ teaspoon ground black pepper

Preheat the oven to 375°F. In a small bowl, toss the chickpeas with the oil, coriander, curry powder, chili flakes, salt, and pepper. Arrange in a single layer on a baking sheet. Bake for 45 minutes, or until crisp and slightly browned. Serve warm or allow to cool.

Makes 4 (¼-cup) servings

Per serving: **110 calories, 6 g protein, 17 g carbohydrates, 3 g fat (0 g saturated), 0 mg cholesterol, 5 g fiber, 150 mg sodium**

Grocery Store Tour

Chickpeas

Also known as garbanzo beans, these legumes are a cost-effective way to enjoy healthy protein. If you buy canned chickpeas, be sure to rinse them well before eating, as they can be loaded with sodium. Dried chickpeas are even cheaper and can be found in packages or bulk bins at the grocery store. They do require extra time to soak and cook, but the flavor and texture are better. Half a cup of cooked chickpeas has 134 calories, 7 grams of protein, and 6 grams of fiber.

VEGETARIAN CURRY STEW

This fragrant and robust stew is a favorite when the weather turns cool. Serve it hot over steaming brown rice or whole grains for a hearty meal. You can also experiment with different beans or try substituting lentils or tofu.

1 tablespoon olive oil

2 cups finely chopped red onions

2 tablespoons finely chopped, peeled fresh ginger

1 tablespoon minced garlic

1 cup diced fire-roasted tomatoes or chopped, seeded, peeled fresh tomatoes, or tomato sauce

1 tablespoon ground coriander

1 tablespoon ground cumin

½ teaspoon ground cardamom

¼ teaspoon ground cinnamon

3 cups fat-free, low-sodium vegetable or chicken broth

1 (12-ounce) sweet potato, peeled and cut into ½" cubes (about 2 cups)

1 cup cooked black beans (see note)

1 cup cooked chickpeas (see note)

Salt and pepper, to taste

⅓ cup chopped fresh cilantro, without stems

Fresh lime wedges

In a large, heavy pot, heat the oil over medium heat. Add the onions and cook, stirring occasionally, for about 10 minutes, or until tender but not brown. Add the ginger and garlic and cook for about 1 minute, or until fragrant. Do not brown the garlic.

Add the tomatoes and simmer for 5 minutes. Add the coriander, cumin, cardamom, and cinnamon and cook for about 1 minute, or until very fragrant. Add the broth and bring to a boil. Stir in the sweet potato and simmer for about 4 minutes. Add the beans and chickpeas and simmer for about 5 minutes, or until cooked through. Season with salt and pepper. Serve hot, sprinkled with cilantro and a squeeze of lime juice.

Note: For chicken curry, add 1 pound boneless, skinless chicken breasts, cut into ½" cubes, in place of the beans and chickpeas.

Makes 8 (1-cup) servings

Per serving: 160 calories, 6 g protein, 28 g carbohydrates, 2 g fat (0 g saturated), 0 mg cholesterol, 6 g fiber, 250 mg sodium

TANGY TURKEY WRAP

This protein-packed turkey salad makes a satisfying lunch and is also delicious on top of salad greens, without the wrap. If you prefer, boneless, skinless chicken breast can be substituted for the turkey.

⅓ cup plain, fat-free Greek-style yogurt

¼ cup low-fat mayonnaise

2 tablespoons chutney

1 teaspoon lime juice

1 teaspoon curry powder

½ teaspoon ground cumin

¼ teaspoon ground coriander

1 tablespoon olive oil

¾ cup diced yellow onion

1 teaspoon chopped garlic

1 pound boneless, skinless turkey breast, cut in short, ½"-thick strips

½ teaspoon salt

½ cup chopped prunes or dried berries (such as cranberries)

3 tablespoons fresh cilantro, chopped

6 (7") whole grain tortillas (I use La Tortilla Factory)

In a medium mixing bowl, combine the yogurt, mayonnaise, chutney, lime juice, curry powder, cumin, and coriander. Set aside.

In a nonstick skillet, heat the oil over medium-high heat. Add the onion and cook for about 4 minutes, or until soft and just beginning to brown. Add the garlic and cook for 1 minute longer. Don't allow the garlic to brown. Add the turkey and cook, stirring frequently, for about 4 minutes, or until just cooked through. Remove from the heat and season with the salt. Add the turkey mixture to the dressing in the mixing bowl. Add the prunes and cilantro. Stir to combine. There will be approximately 3 cups of turkey salad.

Place about ½ cup turkey salad on a warmed tortilla. Roll it up, burrito style, and serve immediately.

Makes 6 small wraps

Per serving: 270 calories, 23 g protein, 32 g carbohydrates, 6 g fat (2 g saturated), 33 mg cholesterol, 11 g fiber, 350 mg sodium

GARLICKY POACHED CHICKEN BREASTS WITH GINGER AND ONION

Poaching in water is a wonderful way to cook protein without adding fat. In this recipe, chicken breasts are poached in a flavorful, aromatic broth. You can substitute turkey tenders for the chicken, but if you do, be sure to cut the cooking time in half. Try pairing this dish with brown rice and a salad for a complete meal.

4 cups fat-free, low-sodium chicken broth

10 baby carrots, quartered lengthwise

1 medium stalk celery, thinly sliced on the diagonal

½ medium yellow onion, finely chopped

2 tablespoons chopped fresh ginger

1 tablespoon chopped garlic

¼ cup low-sodium soy sauce

4 boneless, skinless chicken breasts (about 1¼ pounds)

4 ounces trimmed snow peas

2 tablespoons chopped chives or scallions

In a large saucepan, heat the broth to boiling. Add the carrots, celery, onion, ginger, garlic, and soy sauce. Reduce the heat, cover, and simmer for 10 minutes.

Add the chicken breasts to the simmering broth over medium-low heat. When the broth returns to a boil, turn the chicken. Simmer for 3 minutes, then add the snow peas. Simmer for about 3 minutes longer, or until the chicken is just cooked.

Transfer the chicken and vegetables to large, shallow serving bowls. Ladle the broth over the chicken and garnish with chives or scallions.

Makes 4 servings

Per serving: 200 calories, 36 g protein, 9 g carbohydrates, 2 g fat (less than 1 g saturated), 80 mg cholesterol, 3 g fiber, 445 mg sodium

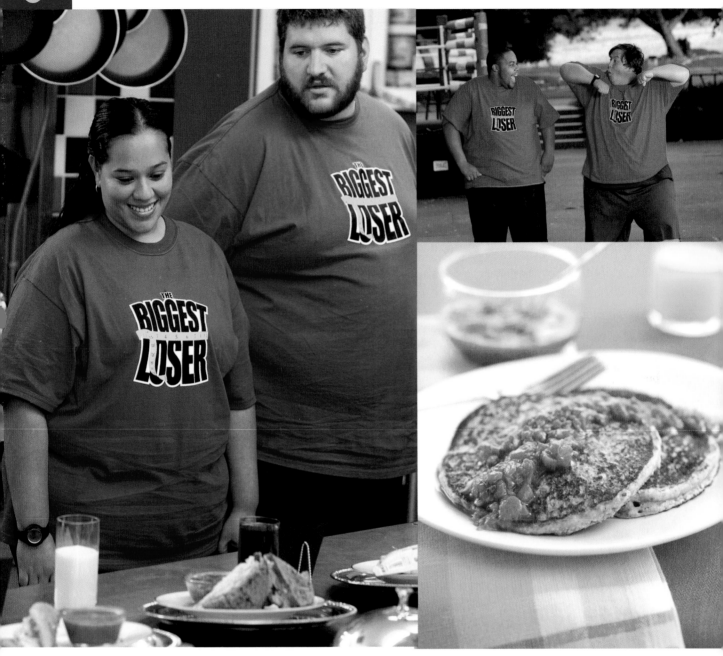

Don't Go Against the Grain

"The first thing I noticed when I got to the ranch," says Amanda Arlauskas of Season 8, "was how different the food was. I've never eaten a lot of healthy food. But our refrigerators and cabinets are stocked with a lot of really good food that I've learned to like." *Biggest Loser* contestants meet all kinds of new vegetables and fruits in the ranch kitchen, but they *really* get to know the world of whole grains. In the contestants' preranch existence, carbohydrates were often consumed in the form of doughnuts and hamburger buns. At the ranch, they're introduced to barley, oats, lentils, and bulgur. They eat high-fiber cereals and breads and bake whole wheat pitas to make healthy snacks.

The contestants quickly learn that the processed carbs found in many of the breads and pastas they

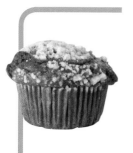

SWAP A BRAN MUFFIN FOR AN ENGLISH MUFFIN.

This swap may sound counterintuitive, but check the labels and you'll find that many of the whole grain English muffins now available exceed the fiber per serving found in most ready-made bran muffins, and are generally much lower in calories.

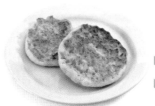

of the kernel is the endosperm. After a grain has been processed, the endosperm is all that remains. It still contains protein and carbohydrate, but the precious fiber and most of the nutrients have been stripped away.

When you read the labels of packaged carbohydrates, watch out for the term *enriched*. It usually indicates that a food like bread or pasta has been made with processed flour, meaning the nutrients have been removed and then replaced synthetically. Foods made with enriched flours are also typically high in carbs and low in fiber.

Meet the Grains

The whole grain family includes barley, corn, oats, quinoa, rice, and wheat. These are all great sources of protein, B vitamins, antioxidants, and fiber. They're also loaded with antiaging benefits.

Barley

Hulled barley, also known as barley groats, is the least processed form of the grain. Only the outermost hull is removed. Pearl barley, on the other hand, is stripped of both the hull and the nutritious bran layer. Hulled barley takes slightly longer to cook but has an interesting flavor and texture and contains more fiber and nutrients.

Corn

Because the germ has not been removed, stone-ground cornmeal is much more nutritious than ordinary cornmeal. The preservation of the germ increases the fat content slightly and decreases the shelf life of this grain. Stone-ground cornmeal is available in most heath food stores and should be kept refrigerated.

Oats

Typically thought of as a breakfast food, oats are a nutritional powerhouse. Oats help maintain bone strength and promote heart health, and they pos-

Spice It Up!

Though you should keep a close eye on your sodium intake, some foods are really enhanced by small sprinkle of salt. I love the freshness that citrus brings to salt flavor and keep my own blend of citrus salt on hand. You can make it by mixing ½ cup of sea salt or kosher salt with 2 tablespoons of fresh citrus zest (lemon, lime, or orange). Spread on a cookie sheet and bake at 200°F for 2 hours, or until the zest is dry. Blend zest in a food processor until evenly mixed, and store in airtight container or resealable plastic bag.

sess a unique fiber that binds with cholesterol in the intestinal tract and helps reduce unhealthy (LDL) cholesterol levels. Because it's an insoluble fiber, it also slows the release of glucose into the bloodstream, improving blood sugar control and curbing your carb cravings.

Quinoa

Quinoa is an ancient grain that originated in South America. It is a good source of protein, fiber, iron, and magnesium and is gluten free, so it can be eaten by people with wheat allergies or sensitivities. Quinoa has a delicious, nutty flavor and a hearty texture that adds bulk to any meal.

Rice

White rice has been processed to remove the husk, bran, and germ, which also removes most nutrients and fiber. Brown rice is higher in vitamins and fiber than white rice. Wild rice is grainlike but is technically a grass. It's high in protein, fiber, and B vitamins and is gluten free.

Wheat

Wheat is considered the "bread grain," because it contains gluten-forming proteins that give structure

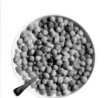

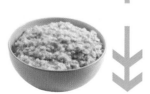

SWAP SUGARY CEREALS FOR WHOLE GRAINS.

The slow release of energy from complex carbs will help you feel full longer while keeping your blood sugar steady and your energy revved. Choose a cereal that has at least 5 grams of fiber and *no more than* 5 grams of sugar per serving. Try the Hi-Pro Vanilla Breakfast Grains recipe on page 85.

to baked goods. Wheat flour is the result of grinding wheat kernels. Though refined wheat flour is a primary ingredient in countless "empty-calorie" foods, its unrefined counterparts are loaded with nutrients. Bulgur (also spelled bulghur) is made from whole wheat berries that are steamed, partially debranned, dried, and crushed or cracked. A meal with bulgur also provides protein and fiber. The result is steady energy that lasts long beyond mealtime. Available in coarse, medium, and fine grinds, bulgur is a staple in the Middle Eastern diet. Usually seen on the lunch or dinner table, it's also an ideal breakfast grain.

Below, you'll find the fiber content of common whole grains.

GRAIN (¼ CUP UNCOOKED)	FIBER (GRAMS)
Barley	8
Bulgur	6
Wheat germ	4
Whole wheat couscous	4
Quinoa	3
Wild rice	3
Cream of wheat	2
High-fiber cornmeal	2
Rolled oats	2

On *The Biggest Loser* nutrition plan, you eat two servings of whole grains daily.

Bread

Serving size: *2 slices bread, preferably "light"; 1 whole grain bun or roll; 2 light Wasa flatbreads; 1 whole wheat flour tortilla*

Choose breads with 3 grams of fiber or more per serving. Always read the labels when you're in the bread aisle of the grocery store. Make sure the first

SWAP NOODLES FOR SAUCE AND VEGGIES.

The next time you eat pasta, make it more about the sauce than about the noodles— you'll get to enjoy the same portion of food, but with many fewer calories. If you're dining out, ask about this option or try the Greek-Style Pasta with Fire-Roasted Tomato Sauce and Crumbled Feta Cheese recipe on page 67.

SWAP OUT EMPTY-CALORIE WHITE FLOUR WAFFLES AND PANCAKES.

Instead of filling up on pancakes and waffles with high-calorie syrup, start your day with omega-3-rich flaxseed, which will keep you feeling fuller longer and contains heart-healthy fats. Sprinkle flaxseed on your favorite whole grain cereal or try the Golden Flaxjacks recipe on page 104.

ingredient listed is "whole wheat" or "whole grain."
If "wheat flour" is the first ingredient, it usually
means that the product is made from enriched white
flour with some whole wheat added.

Choose these to lose: Ezekiel bread, high-fiber
bread (choose brands with around 45 calories per
slice), Wasa flatbreads, whole grain bread, whole
wheat buns, whole wheat dinner rolls, whole wheat
pitas, and whole wheat tortillas.

Grains

Serving size: *1 cup cooked*

Avoid most packaged, ready-to-eat breakfast cereals. These tend to be highly processed and loaded
with added sugar. Go for cereals that contain
5 grams of fiber or more, and be cautious of sugar
content. Although all cereals will naturally contain
some sugar, avoid cereals that have 5 grams of
sugar or more per serving.

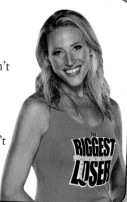

Tara Costa, Season 7 Finalist

You need to eat! You can't
lose weight if you don't
eat. Also, read all the
ingredients on food
packages, and if you don't
know what something is,
don't put it in your mouth.

Choose these to lose: Barley, brown rice, bulgur,
corn grits, couscous, cream of rice, cream of wheat,
millet, oat bran, quinoa, rolled oats, whole wheat
cereal, whole wheat pasta, and wild rice.

What to Avoid: The Bad Carbs

If you're trying to lose weight but find yourself constantly battling carb cravings, it could be partially

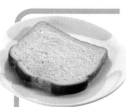

SWAP WHITE BREAD FOR WHOLE WHEAT.

Not only do dense whole grain breads have more antioxidants and fiber per
slice, but their textures and flavors make them much tastier, too.
Be sure to use this swap wherever you use bread—in French
toast, croutons, breading, and stuffing.

that your food choices are sabotaging your efforts. Eating some refined carbohydrates can stimulate your appetite and make you even hungrier. These choices, which include white bread and many packaged bakery products, are stripped of fiber content and turn to sugar quickly in the body.

Some examples of carbs to avoid:

- White bread
- White pasta
- White potatoes
- Pastries
- Doughnuts
- Cookies, snack cakes, pies, and other sugary baked goods
- Candy and candy bars
- Potato chips and other packaged and fried snacks

Why do these foods give you that irresistible urge to raid the fridge or pantry? Because the sugar and refined starches they contain cause your blood sugar to soar. In response to that sugar surge, your body churns out the hormone insulin—so much that it drives your blood sugar below where it was before you ate anything. When blood sugar is that low, you feel tired and hungry and in need of another quick pick-me-up—often in the form of something sweet. These ups and downs, coupled with the wrong food choices, can wreak havoc on your weight-loss efforts. When a food contains both fat and sugar, as many of the foods listed here do, it can be downright addictive, since many of us crave the tastes of fat and sugar.

Liz Young, Season 8

My husband had bypass surgery about 4 years ago. It was very unexpected. One day he went to the hospital thinking he had an ear infection, and he ended up having a quadruple bypass. And I'm very sure that it was partly due to the way I cook. We weren't eating as healthfully as we probably should have been. I'm from the South, and I grew up on fried chicken, mashed potatoes, homemade biscuits, and cornbread. What's healthy about that? Nothing.

That's one of the most important things I'm learning from *The Biggest Loser*: how to cook properly and how to combine the right foods. I'm working on finding that balance. Nutrition is definitely going to play a huge role in my weight-loss journey. But I'm ready for the change.

Steel-Cut Oats

These oats are made from the inner part of the oat kernel, and unlike flattened rolled oats, they're roughly cut into small, nubby pieces. They take a bit longer to cook than rolled oats, but their flavor and texture are worth it. I save money by purchasing these oats from the bulk bin, and I keep them handy in a canister on my kitchen counter. A half cup of dry steel-cut oats contains about 140 calories, 6 grams of protein, and 4 grams of fiber. The oats roughly double in size during cooking. You can cook several servings at a time and refrigerate unused portions for several days.

Polenta

Polenta is a paste or powder made of ground dried corn and can be prepared on its own or combined with other ingredients. Polenta and cornmeal are used interchangeably in many recipes—the difference between the two is the size of the grind, and consequently the price. Cornmeal can be ground to a fine, medium, or coarse texture. Cornbread and muffins often call for a fine grind, which is similar to the texture of flour. Polenta requires a medium or coarse grind. Try Cornbread Stuffing with Sausage and Prunes on page 112.

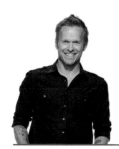

Trainer Tip: BOB HARPER

It's possible to make even pizza healthy using whole grains. Start by using whole wheat dough, and then add low-fat mozzarella cheese. Top with heaps of nutrient-rich vegetables, a lean protein such as chicken or shrimp, and even some fruit. Pears, apples, and pineapple add a touch of sweetness and bring out the flavors in the veggies.

GOLDEN FLAXJACKS

Whole grains add texture and flavor to any recipe, and flaxseed contains heart-healthy omega-3s. Cook your flaxjacks over moderate heat so they don't burn; the flaxseed makes them brown more quickly. Serve hot with Strawberry Fruit Spread (page 128) or low-calorie syrup.

1 cup whole wheat flour

½ cup stone-ground cornmeal

2 tablespoons wheat bran or oat bran

2 tablespoons flaxseed meal (see note)

2 teaspoons baking powder

½ teaspoon salt

2 large egg whites

1¾ cups fat-free or 1% milk

2 tablespoons olive oil or canola oil

½ teaspoon pure vanilla extract

In a large mixing bowl, combine the flour, cornmeal, bran, flaxseed meal, baking powder, and salt. Set aside.

In a small mixing bowl or blender, whisk together the egg whites, milk, oil, and vanilla until smooth. Make a well in the center of the dry ingredients. Pour the liquid mixture into the well and stir just until combined. Allow the batter to stand for about 30 minutes or overnight in the refrigerator. Add more milk, if needed, to obtain batter the consistency of thick cream.

Heat a nonstick griddle or nonstick skillet (coated with cooking spray if necessary) to medium heat. For each flaxjack, pour a scant ¼ cup of batter onto the griddle. Cook until the flaxjacks are puffed and dry around the edges. Turn and cook the other side until golden brown.

Note: If you can't find flaxseed meal, you can grind whole flaxseeds yourself in a spice grinder or clean coffee grinder. Grind to the consistency of cornmeal. Four teaspoons of whole flaxseeds yield approximately 2 tablespoons of flaxseed meal.

Makes 8 servings of 2 (4") flaxjacks

Per serving: 160 calories, 6 g protein, 23 g carbohydrates, 5 g fat (1 g saturated), 0 mg cholesterol, 4 g fiber, 320 mg sodium

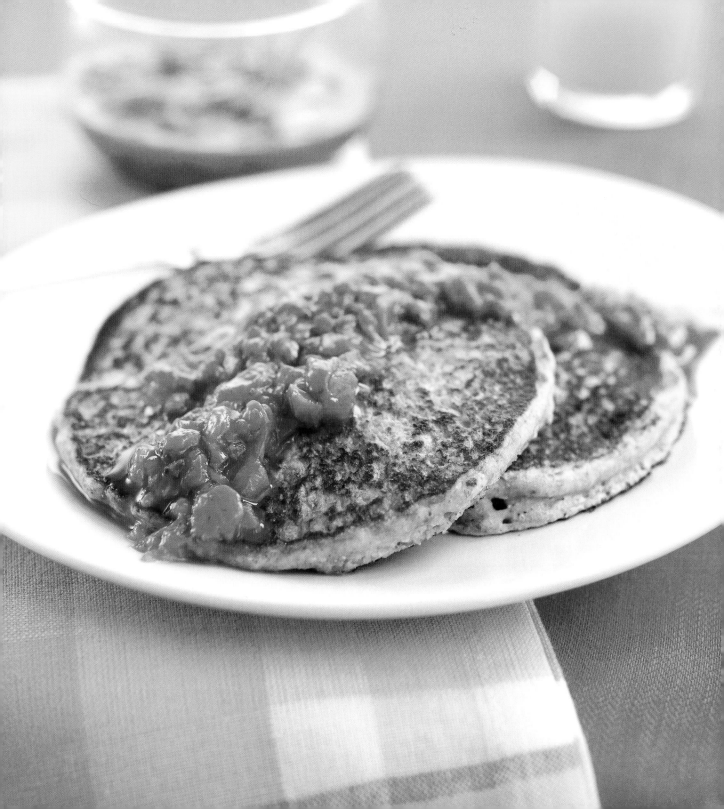

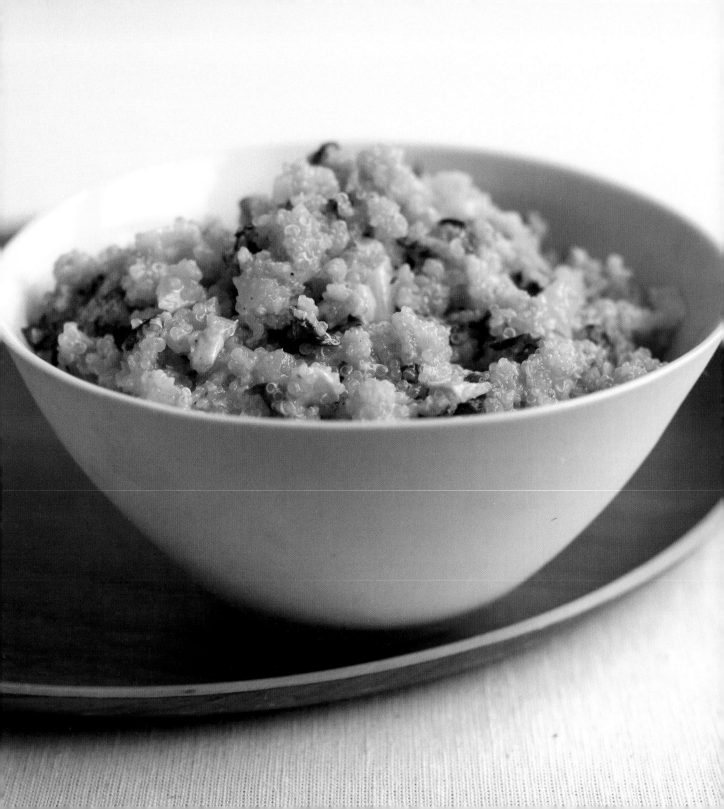

QUINOA WITH SPINACH AND CHEESE

This high-protein Incan grain is truly an ancient treasure. It can be simmered in milk for a breakfast or dessert dish, or, as prepared here, it can be cooked in broth for a warm pilaf or a delicious cold salad.

- 2 teaspoons olive oil
- 1 cup diced onion
- ¼ cup diced celery
- 1 teaspoon minced garlic
- 1 cup quinoa, rinsed well
- 2 cups fat-free, low-sodium chicken broth or vegetable broth
- 2 cups chopped spinach or kale or Swiss chard
- ½ cup chopped mushrooms
- ¼ cup grated Parmesan cheese
- ½ teaspoon salt
- ¼ teaspoon ground black pepper

In a saucepan, heat the oil over medium heat. Add the onion and celery and cook for about 5 minutes, or until soft and translucent. Add the garlic and quinoa and cook for about 1 minute longer, stirring occasionally. Do not brown the garlic. Add the broth and bring to a boil.

Reduce the heat to low and simmer for about 12 minutes; the mixture will be brothy and the quinoa almost done. Stir in the spinach and mushrooms and simmer for 2 minutes longer, or until the quinoa grains have turned from white to transparent. Add the cheese. Season with the salt and pepper. Serve hot.

Makes 6 (about ¾-cup) servings

Per serving: 160 calories, 7 g protein, 24 g carbohydrates, 4 g fat (1 g saturated), 5 mg cholesterol, 2 g fiber, 320 mg sodium

Grocery Store Tour

Quinoa

You can find quinoa in the rice and pasta aisle of most grocery stores, or in a bulk bin at your local natural foods store. Half a cup of cooked quinoa contains 110 calories, 8 grams of protein, and 5 grams of fiber.

NICOLE AND DAMIEN'S SWEET GRILLED CHEESE SANDWICH

This yummy, easy snack is perfect for sharing with a friend or, in the case of Season 7 lovebirds Nicole Brewer and Damien Gurganious, your spouse!

2 slices low-fat provolone or Swiss cheese

2 slices Ezekiel cinnamon raisin bread

Spray a small nonstick skillet with cooking oil spray. Place the cheese between the slices of bread. Heat the pan over medium-high heat and add the sandwich. Gently press down with a spatula once or twice during grilling. When one side is golden, turn the sandwich over and cook until golden brown.

Cut the sandwich in half and serve immediately.

Makes 1 sandwich

Per ½ sandwich: **120 calories, 8 g protein, 20 g carbohydrates, 2 g fat (less than 1 g saturated), 5 mg cholesterol, 2 g fiber, 270 mg sodium**

Alexandra White, Season 8

I've been overweight my entire life. Growing up, I think we used food in the wrong way—you don't have to celebrate every occasion with food. Now I'm having fun experimenting with all the new healthy foods I've learned about at the ranch. And it all tastes great!

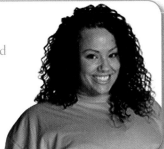

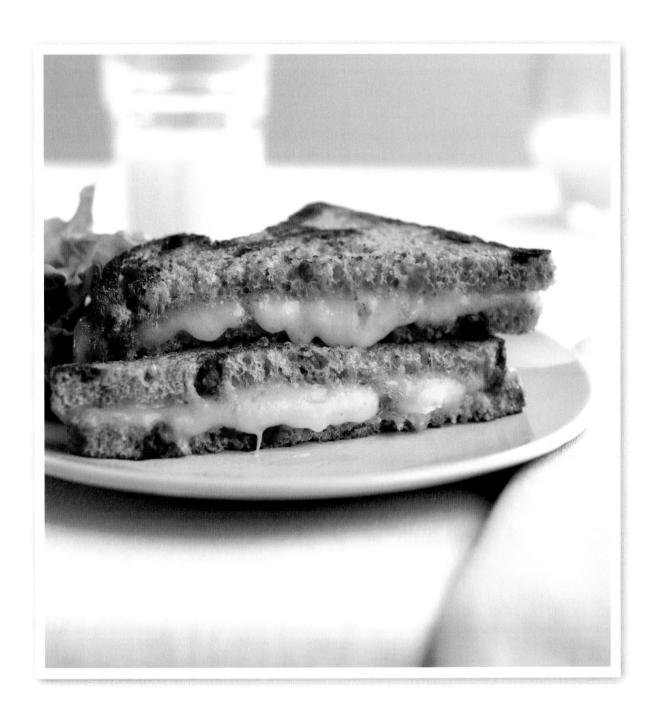

ASIAN WILD RICE SAUTÉ

I used to prepare this side dish in a restaurant in the Loire Valley of France where the chef loved to combine French cuisine with Asian influences. Though the flavors are complex, the preparation is amazingly simple.

2 teaspoons olive oil

¾ cup finely chopped yellow bell pepper

¾ cup finely chopped red bell pepper

2 cups cooked wild rice

½ teaspoon ground cinnamon

½ teaspoon salt

2 tablespoons chopped fresh cilantro

In a nonstick skillet, heat the oil. Add the bell peppers and cook for a few minutes, until softened but not mushy. Add the wild rice. Stir and cook for a few minutes, or until the rice is just heated through. Add the cinnamon, salt, and cilantro. Stir well and serve immediately.

Makes 4 (¾-cup) servings

Per serving: 120 calories, 4 g protein, 21 g carbohydrates, 2 g fat (0 g saturated), 0 mg cholesterol, 3 g fiber, 300 mg sodium

Grocery Store Tour

Wild Rice

Wild rice is actually a cereal grass, though it looks very much like a dark-colored rice. It can be used the same ways as other rice—as a side dish, in soups, or mixed with vegetables. If you use it often, it's a good idea to buy it in bulk, because it is a bit pricier than white rice. Half a cup contains 82 calories, 3 grams of protein, and 3 grams of fiber.

BUTTERMILK CORNBREAD

This easy recipe can be transformed into a scrumptious, savory dressing for your Thanksgiving turkey or a special meal.

1 cup yellow whole grain cornmeal

¾ cup whole wheat flour

2 teaspoons baking powder

1 teaspoon salt

¼ teaspoon baking soda

1 cup 1% buttermilk

2 tablespoons light olive oil

2 eggs

2 tablespoons xylitol or dark honey or agave nectar

Preheat the oven to 400°F. Lightly coat an 8" × 8" baking pan with cooking spray. Set aside.

In a medium mixing bowl, combine the cornmeal, flour, baking powder, salt, and baking soda. Set aside.

In a small mixing bowl, whisk together the buttermilk, oil, eggs, and xylitol. Pour the liquid ingredients into the dry ingredients and mix with a fork, just until smooth. Pour into the prepared baking pan and bake for 18 minutes, or until a toothpick inserted near the center comes out clean. Cool on a wire rack.

To make dry cornbread cubes: Preheat the oven to 400°F. Cut the cornbread into ½" cubes. Place the cubes on baking sheets and bake for 5 to 7 minutes, or until lightly browned. Cool on a wire rack. There will be about 8 cups of cubed cornbread.

Makes 9 (2½"-square) servings

Per serving: 150 calories, 5 g protein, 28 g carbohydrates, 2 g fat (less than 1 g saturated), 50 mg cholesterol, 3 g fiber, 450 mg sodium

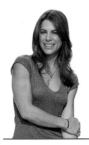

Trainer Tip: JILLIAN MICHAELS

We've known for many years that the fiber in whole grains aids in digestive health. Recent studies have shown that eating more whole grains may also reduce the risk of heart disease, cancer, and diabetes. So get a great start on the day by eating whole grain carbohydrates.

CORNBREAD STUFFING WITH SAUSAGE AND PRUNES

This scrumptious stuffing is fancy enough for a special occasion but so delicious that it's bound to become a mainstay on your dinner table. And unlike most stuffing, it's as rich in health benefits as it is in flavor.

8 cups toasted Buttermilk Cornbread cubes (page 111; see note)

8 ounces (about 2 links) lean turkey Italian sausage

1 tablespoon olive oil

2 cups chopped onions

½ cup chopped celery

½ cup chopped carrot

1 teaspoon chopped garlic

1 cup coarsely chopped prunes

1 teaspoon dried thyme

1 teaspoon dried sage

½ teaspoon dried marjoram

2 cups fat-free, low-sodium chicken broth

3 tablespoons chopped fresh parsley

1 teaspoon salt

½ teaspoon ground pepper

2 large eggs, lightly beaten

Preheat the oven to 325°F. Place the toasted bread cubes in a large bowl and set aside.

In a small nonstick skillet, cook the sausage over medium-high heat until brown and cooked through. Drain well, crumble, and set aside.

In a large nonstick skillet, heat the oil over medium heat. Stir in the onions, celery, and carrot, and cook for 5 minutes, stirring frequently. Add the garlic and cook for 1 minute longer, but don't allow the garlic to brown. Stir in the sausage, prunes, thyme, sage, marjoram, and ½ cup of the broth and bring to a boil. Reduce the heat and simmer for 3 minutes. Remove from the heat. Pour the vegetable mixture over the cornbread. Add the parsley and stir well. Season with the salt and pepper. (The stuffing may be prepared to this stage a day ahead and refrigerated, covered, in the mixing bowl.)

Transfer the stuffing to the prepared baking dish. Combine the eggs and the remaining 1½ cups broth and pour over the cornbread mixture, tossing well. Cover the baking dish with foil. Bake the stuffing for 25 minutes. Remove the foil. Turn the oven up to 375°F and bake the stuffing for about 10 minutes longer, or until the top begins to brown.

Makes 16 (about ½-cup) servings

Per serving: 150 calories, 7 g protein, 22 g carbohydrates, 4 g fat (1 g saturated), 65 mg cholesterol, 3 g fiber, 400 mg sodium

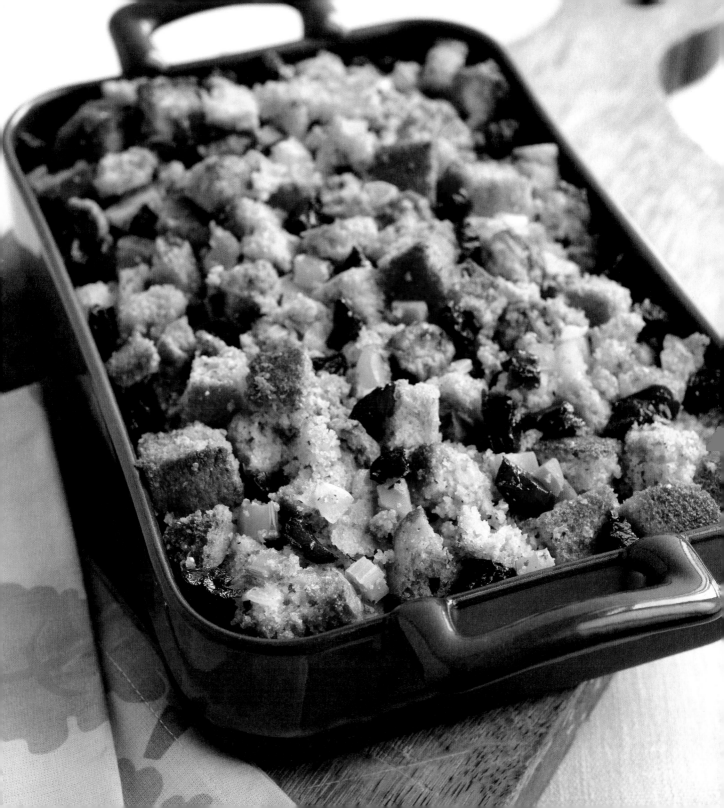

SUNRISE POLENTA WITH VANILLA AND BLUEBERRIES

What better way to greet a brisk fall or winter day than with a steaming bowl of hot cereal? This is a great basic recipe to experiment with—you can stir in your favorite fruit, nuts, spices, or fat-free milk. It's also delicious with the Strawberry Fruit Spread on page 128.

1 cup stone-ground cornmeal

4 cups unsweetened vanilla Almond Breeze nondairy beverage

½ teaspoon pure vanilla extract

1 cup fresh blueberries

In a 2-quart saucepan, heat the cornmeal over medium heat, stirring constantly, for about 3 minutes, or until lightly toasted. Remove from the heat and carefully pour in the Almond Breeze.

Return to the heat and bring to a simmer. Reduce the heat to low and simmer, stirring regularly, for about 10 minutes, or until the cereal is thickened and creamy.

Remove from the heat and allow to stand for 5 minutes. Stir in the vanilla and berries. Serve immediately.

Makes 6 servings

Per serving: 110 calories, 3 g protein, 19 g carbohydrates, 2 g fat (0 g saturated), 0 mg cholesterol, 3 g fiber, 120 mg sodium

Spice It Up!

For a delicious, sugar-free way to satisfy a sweet tooth, sprinkle on some spice! Pumpkin pie spice—which is used in many holiday dessert recipes—is wonderfully aromatic and delivers a punch of sweet, spicy flavor. Try making your own by combining 2 tablespoons ground cinnamon, 1 tablespoon ground ginger, 1 tablespoon cloves, and 2 teaspoons ground nutmeg. Stir to combine and store in an airtight jar or zip-top bag. Add ½ teaspoon of this delicious blend to your hot cereal, yogurt, or smoothie.

CONFETTI COUSCOUS

Couscous, which is made from ground wheat, is a staple in North African cuisine and is actually considered a type of pasta. This sweet, spicy couscous is delicious on its own or can be paired with a chicken breast for a meal. One cup of dry couscous yields about 1 cup cooked. Be sure to buy whole wheat couscous.

½ cup raisins

½ cup finely chopped white onion

½ cup finely chopped red bell pepper

½ cup finely chopped yellow bell pepper

2 teaspoons olive oil

1 tablespoon finely chopped garlic

3 cups cooked whole wheat couscous, prepared according to package directions

1 cup cooked chickpeas (if using canned, rinse well)

¼ cup chopped fresh cilantro

2 teaspoons fresh lemon peel

1 teaspoon ground cinnamon

¾ teaspoon ground dry turmeric

¾ teaspoon salt

Soak the raisins in ½ cup warm water and set aside.

In a nonstick skillet, cook the onion and bell peppers in the oil until just soft. Add the garlic and cook just until fragrant. Transfer to a mixing bowl. Add the couscous, chickpeas, cilantro, lemon peel, cinnamon, turmeric, and salt to the bowl. Toss well and serve chilled or at room temperature.

Makes 8 servings

Per serving: 150 calories, 5 g protein, 29 g carbohydrates, 2 g fat (0 g saturated), 0 mg cholesterol, 5 g fiber, 230 mg sodium

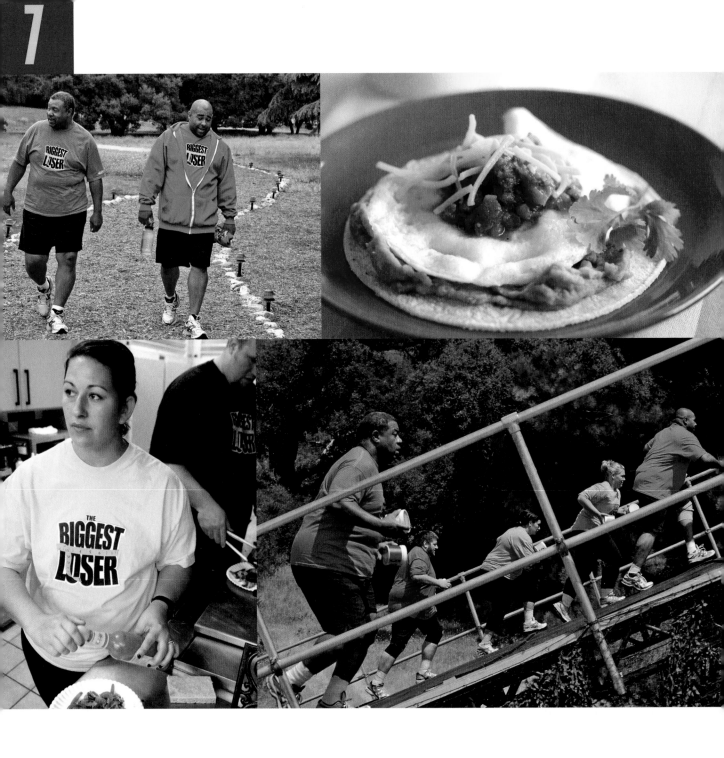

Fat Can Help You Get Thin

Growing up in a family of six, Season 8 contestant Dina Mercado remembers that her family life revolved around celebrations—and eating. "We always celebrated with food, and remember, the last three letters of *celebrate* spell *ate*," she says. Dina celebrated her way up to 243 pounds on her 5-foot-5 frame. And even worse, many of the traditional Mexican foods her family cooked were prepared with lard and oil and were often fried.

A lot of the contestants arrive on the ranch with a near addiction to another dangerous fat: butter. Rebecca Meyer of Season 8 used to fry her eggs in butter and use as much as *half a stick* for her grilled cheese sandwiches. "No more!" she says. "I am singing the praises of olive oil. I use a small amount to sauté chicken, and if I want the taste of butter, I just spray on a little butter substitute. I'm satisfied with

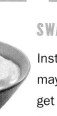

SWAP MAYO FOR AVOCADO.

Instead of slathering your next sandwich with a tablespoon of mayo, try spreading on a few thin slices of avocado. You'll still get the satisfaction of rich flavor and creamy texture, but with fewer calories and the benefit of *good* fats.

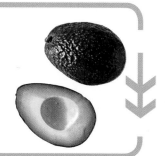

the flavors and don't need all that other unhealthy stuff."

For *Biggest Loser* contestants, learning to cook foods through healthier methods such as grilling and steaming; using good, heart-healthy fats such as olive oil; and adding herbs and spices (not unhealthy fats) for flavor leads not only to better eating habits but also to rejuvenated tastebuds. "The food on the ranch makes me feel much healthier and more satisfied," says Alexandra White of Season 8. In the following pages, you'll learn that just as not all calories are created equal, not all fats are, either. In fact, it's important to incorporate healthy fats into your calorie budget. It's just a matter of swapping bad for good, and, as always, moderation is key.

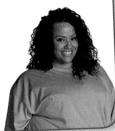

Alexandra White, Season 8

I used to be a big fan of ice cream, but now I make my own version by pureeing frozen strawberries with half a cup of fat-free milk. It's delicious!

Fat Facts

Fad diets come and go. When America declared war on fat, hundreds of fat-free food products flooded the market, because so many people were convinced that fat was the enemy of weight loss.

SWAP FRUIT FOR FRUIT *AND* NUTS.

A piece of fruit has long been considered a healthy snack. But add a few nuts to the mix and you have a *great* healthy snack. A few dry-roasted nuts (almonds, walnuts, or cashews) not only provides the feeling of satiety that their good fats deliver (so you'll feel full longer), but also slows the release of blood sugar for sustained energy—and they taste great! Some sample snack ideas: One medium apple and 2 tablespoons of walnuts (150 calories) or one wedge of cantaloupe plus 2 tablespoons of almonds (140 calories). For a satisfying dish that incorporates fruit and nuts, try the Nutty Waldorf Salad recipe on page 133.

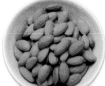

Grocery Store Tour

Olive Oil

Olive oil is a heart-healthy fat that contains antioxidants and helps increase your HDL ("good") cholesterol. Virgin or extra-virgin olive oil contains no refined oils or chemicals. Olive oil can be expensive and is calorie dense, so a little goes a long way. A good method of avoiding waste *and* extra calories is to buy your own pump bottle and fill it with olive oil. Spray just a little oil to coat your pans when cooking.

Avocado

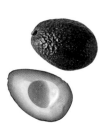

The luscious green color of the avocado tells us it contains a plant chemical called lutein, which helps to promote eye health. Avocados contain good fats that support heart health, as well. Though most of an avocado's calories come from fat, avocados are rich in flavor and texture, so even a small serving is satisfying. For a delicious new way to eat them, try Spaghetti Squash with Avocado Pesto on page 68.

Almonds

Almonds are always on hand at the ranch. Like other nuts, they are calorie dense, so moderation is key. But their crunchy texture and delicious flavor make them a perfect addition to cereal, yogurt, and salads, and they're excellent paired with a piece of fruit for a snack. Almonds contain fat-soluble vitamins, including vitamin E. Almonds are another great item to buy from bulk bins to save money. Choose raw or dry roasted, unsalted almonds and store in an airtight container in a cool place.

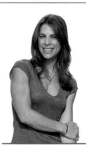

Trainer Tip: JILLIAN MICHAELS

When eating out at a Mexican restaurant, modify your order to make it a healthier meal. Order corn tortillas instead of flour, and veggies instead of refried beans, and ask that the food be cooked in olive oil.

Multiply your total daily calorie budget by 0.25 to see how many calories can come from fat.

$$1,400 \times 0.25 = 350$$

So 350 of your daily calories may come from fat.

One gram of fat contains 9 calories. So simply divide the number of calories from fat that you're allotted each day (in this case, 350) by nine.

$$350 \div 9 = 39$$

In this example, you would consume no more than 39 grams of fat daily.

The easy reference table below shows you the fat values for a range of daily calorie budgets. If your needs aren't reflected below, you can do the math to determine your daily fat intake.

DAILY CALORIE INTAKE	MAXIMUM GRAMS OF TOTAL FAT	MAXIMUM GRAMS OF SATURATED FAT (10% OF DAILY CALORIES)
1,200	33	13
1,300	36	14
1,400	39	16
1,500	42	17
1,600	44	18
1,700	47	19
1,800	50	20
1,900	53	21
2,000	56	22
2,100	58	23
2,200	61	24
2,300	64	26
2,400	67	27
2,500	69	28
2,600	72	29

How to Include Fats in Your Diet

At the top of *The Biggest Loser* food pyramid (page 53) is a 200-calorie budget that's yours to spend on *healthy* extras—not to squander on nutritionally bankrupt foods such as candy, soda, or chips. Sensible, healthy choices for this discretionary calorie budget include the following foods and condiments.

Fats, Oils, and Spreads

Choose these to lose: Olive oil, canola oil, flaxseed oil, or walnut oil for salads, cooking, and baking; reduced-fat and fat-free salad dressings and mayonnaise; avocados; reduced-fat peanut butter and nut butters.

Reduced-Fat Foods

Choose these to lose: reduced-fat or fat-free cheeses, fat-free sour cream.

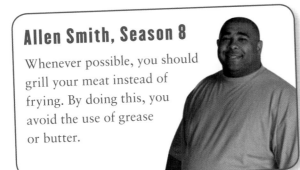

Allen Smith, Season 8

Whenever possible, you should grill your meat instead of frying. By doing this, you avoid the use of grease or butter.

SWAP YOUR REGULAR PAN FOR A NONSTICK VERSION.

One tablespoon of cooking oil has a whopping 120 calories! You'll save big-time if you switch to a nonstick pan with just a small spray of olive oil. For another low-fat method, try the recipe for Halibut Romesco on page 125.

SWAP BUTTER FOR FRUIT SPREAD.

A tablespoon of butter has 100 calories and 11 grams of fat, including 7 grams of saturated fat. The next time you have toast, spread on some no-sugar-added fruit spread for only 40 calories, and get antioxidants to boot! Try the Strawberry Fruit Spread recipe on page 128.

SWAP GRANOLA FOR NUTS.

Granola adds texture as a topping for yogurt or cereal—but many varieties are loaded with sugar, fat, and calories. Sprinkle on a tablespoon of crushed almonds or walnuts instead and get the benefit of heart-healthy omega-3s plus protein with your crunch.

Other

Choose these to lose: nuts and seeds, including flaxseeds; avocado; olives.

Fats to Avoid

When you're trying to lose weight, the most important fats to avoid are animal fats (found in egg yolks, meat products, and full-fat dairy products) and trans fat (found in margarine and foods that contain hydrogenated oils). Not only are both of these fats loaded with calories, but they can also interfere with your body's ability to use good fats that protect you from disease.

One great strategy for eliminating unnecessary fats from your diet is to cook without added fats. Instead of sautéing or pan-frying, try baking, broiling, grilling, poaching, or steaming your food. And when you do use oil, olive oil is the best choice. Remember—just a spray (not a pour) will do to coat your pans.

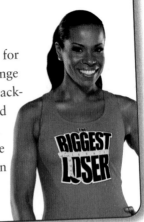

Nicole Brewer, Season 7

I use just the egg whites for omelets now. Also, I cringe now at the thought of packaged foods and prepared foods. I crave fresh and clean foods that I make at home. That way I can control what's in my meals.

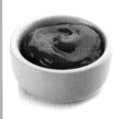

SWAP BAD CONDIMENTS FOR GOOD ONES.

Salad dressings, creamy dips, ketchup, and mayonnaise can quickly add up to hundreds of extra calories. Experiment with different mustards, salsas, low-sugar ketchups and barbecue sauces, and vinegars to add flavor to your food. You'll be amazed at the calorie and fat savings. If you only swapped your ranch dressing for brown mustard, you could save more than 60 calories and 7 grams of fat!

HALIBUT ROMESCO

Cooking in a packet (en papillote) is surprisingly easy and doesn't require added fat. Because the fish and seasonings are sealed in a packet, all of their juices and flavors are trapped inside. The packets can be assembled a few hours ahead of time and popped in the oven just before dinner. An equal weight of shrimp or scallops can also be used in place of the fish.

4 (5-ounce) fillets halibut, salmon, cod, or sole

1 medium red bell pepper, roasted, peeled, and cut into 2" strips

¼ cup minced yellow onion

2 tablespoons slivered almonds, lightly toasted (see note)

2 teaspoons chopped garlic

2 teaspoons lemon juice

½ teaspoon minced chipotle pepper (see note)

½ teaspoon smoked paprika

½ teaspoon salt

½ teaspoon ground black pepper

Fresh chives or scallions, chopped

Preheat the oven to 400°F. Prepare two 15" × 15" squares of parchment paper (see note). Fold one square of parchment in half to create a crease, then open up. Place both fish fillets on one side of the crease, leaving the other side empty. Repeat with the remaining fillets and parchment.

In a small mixing bowl, combine the bell pepper, onion, almonds, garlic, lemon juice, chipotle pepper, paprika, salt, and black pepper. Top each of the fillets with one-quarter of the pepper mixture.

Fold over the empty side of the paper so that it covers the fish; tightly crimp the outer edges together to create a packet. Be sure to seal the packets completely. Place the packets on a baking sheet.

Bake for 10 to 12 minutes, until the fish flakes easily with a fork.

Place each packet on a dinner plate. To serve, slit the packet with a knife, making an X, and fold back the paper. Garnish with chives or scallions.

Notes: To toast nuts in the oven, preheat the oven to 375°F. Place the nuts in a single layer on a baking sheet and bake for 5 to 8 minutes, or until fragrant. Stir the nuts a few times during baking to ensure even browning. To toast on the stovetop, place the nuts in a small skillet over medium heat. Toast, stirring occasionally, for about 2 minutes.

Chipotle peppers, canned in a spicy sauce called adobo, are available at Latin American markets, specialty foods stores, and some supermarkets.

If you don't have parchment paper on hand, you can substitute squares of foil.

Makes 4 servings

Per serving: 190 calories, 31 g protein, 4 g carbohydrates, 5 g fat (less than 1 g saturated), 45 mg cholesterol, 1 g fiber, 230 mg sodium

HUEVOS RANCHEROS

This quick and tasty ranchero sauce is also fabulous with scrambled eggs or tossed with whole grain pasta for a south-of-the-border flair. And my version of Huevos Rancheros is likely to be much lower in calories than what you'll find at your favorite diner!

Ranchero Sauce:

- 2 teaspoons olive oil
- 1 small yellow onion, chopped
- 1 tablespoon chopped garlic
- 1 (14-ounce) can diced fire-roasted tomatoes
- ½ teaspoon ground coriander
- ½ teaspoon ground cumin
- ½ teaspoon dried oregano
- ½ teaspoon salt
- Ground pepper, to taste
- ½ teaspoon dried chipotle powder (optional)
- ¼ cup chopped fresh cilantro

Huevos Rancheros:

- 1 corn tortilla
- 2 tablespoons fat-free refried beans
- 2 egg whites
- 1 tablespoon low-fat Cheddar cheese
- Fresh cilantro

To make the sauce: Heat the oil in a nonstick skillet. Add the onion and cook for about 5 minutes, or until softened. Add the garlic and cook for about 1 minute longer, but don't allow the garlic to brown. Add the tomatoes, coriander, cumin, oregano, salt, pepper, and chipotle powder (if desired) and cook for a few minutes longer.

Carefully transfer the sauce to the jar of a blender or the bowl of a food processor and blend or process briefly. The finished sauce should be a bit chunky. Stir in the cilantro.

To make one serving of Huevos Rancheros: Warm the tortilla and refried beans and set aside.

Coat a small nonstick skillet with cooking spray. Add the egg whites and cook until nearly set, or about 2 minutes. Turn the eggs with a silicone spatula and cook for about 1 minute longer.

Place the tortilla on a plate and top it with the beans. Place the cooked egg whites on the beans. Top with ½ cup hot Ranchero Sauce and garnish with cheese and cilantro.

Makes 4 (½-cup) servings sauce (enough for 4 servings Huevos Rancheros)

Per serving (sauce only): 50 calories, 1 g protein, 6 g carbohydrates, 0 g fat (0 g saturated), 0 mg cholesterol, 2 g fiber, 530 mg sodium

Per serving (Huevos Rancheros): 180 calories, 14 g protein, 24 g carbohydrates, 3 g fat (less than 1 g saturated), 0 mg cholesterol, 4 g fiber, 530 mg sodium

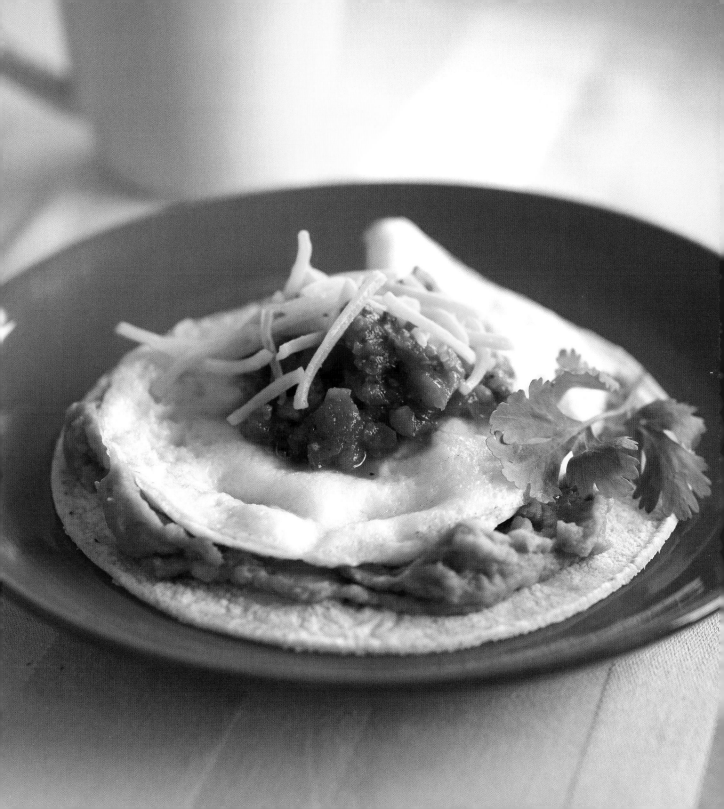

STRAWBERRY FRUIT SPREAD

This sweet, delicious spread is wonderful on whole grain toast or stirred into plain fat-free Greek-style yogurt. It can also add a burst of fruit flavor to your favorite hot cereal.

3 cups fresh strawberries or 12 ounces frozen unsweetened strawberries

1 tablespoon frozen apple juice concentrate

1 teaspoon pure vanilla extract

1 teaspoon ground cinnamon

Place the berries in the bowl of a food processor and pulse until roughly chopped but not pureed. Transfer to a 2-quart saucepan. Add the juice concentrate and bring to a boil over medium-high heat. When the mixture boils, reduce the heat to low. Simmer for about 3 minutes (slightly longer if using frozen berries), stirring occasionally, or until the juices have reduced slightly and the mixture has thickened. Remove from the heat and cool. Stir in the vanilla and cinnamon. Keeps refrigerated for about 2 weeks.

Makes 16 (1-tablespoon) servings (1 cup)

Per serving: 10 calories, 0 g protein, 3 g carbohydrates, 0 g fat (0 g saturated), 0 mg cholesterol, 1 g fiber, 0 mg sodium

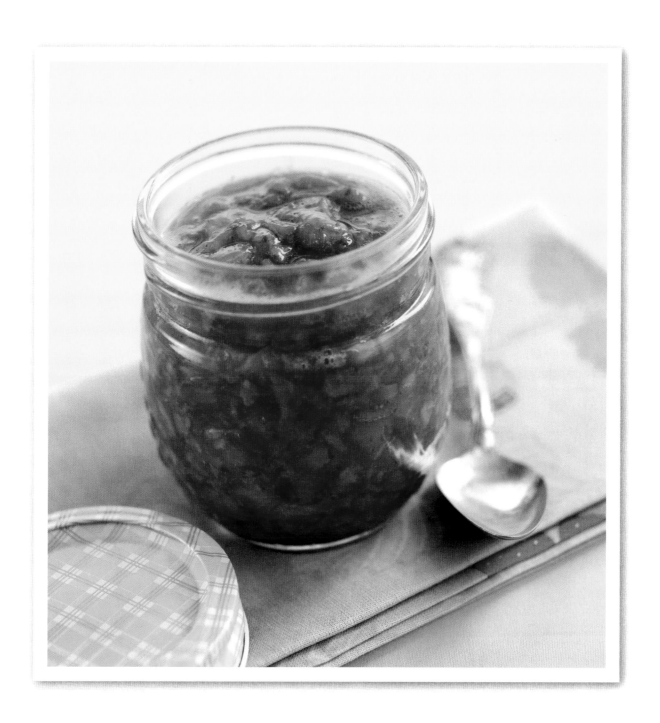

SMOKED SALMON SPREAD

Move over, cream cheese. This light and full-flavored spread is great on a toasted whole grain bagel with tomato slices and capers. It can also be thinned (with more yogurt) and used as a dip. Smoked salmon has a richer color and flavor, but canned pink salmon works well, too.

1 cup (8 ounces) plain, fat-free Greek-style yogurt

¼ cup (2 ounces) low-fat cream cheese

4 ounces finely chopped smoked salmon or drained, canned wild salmon

⅓ cup finely chopped red onion

1 tablespoon prepared horseradish

½ teaspoon lemon juice

½ teaspoon salt

¼ teaspoon ground black pepper

1 tablespoon chopped chives

In a medium mixing bowl, combine the yogurt and cream cheese until smooth. Stir in the salmon, onion, horseradish, lemon juice, salt, pepper, and chives. Refrigerate for at least 1 hour. Stir before serving.

Makes 6 (about ¼" cup) servings

Per serving: 60 calories, 7 g protein, 3 g carbohydrates, 3 g fat (1 g saturated), 10 mg cholesterol, 0 g fiber, 500 mg sodium

SWAP WHITE FOR RED.

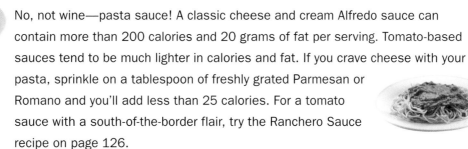

No, not wine—pasta sauce! A classic cheese and cream Alfredo sauce can contain more than 200 calories and 20 grams of fat per serving. Tomato-based sauces tend to be much lighter in calories and fat. If you crave cheese with your pasta, sprinkle on a tablespoon of freshly grated Parmesan or Romano and you'll add less than 25 calories. For a tomato sauce with a south-of-the-border flair, try the Ranchero Sauce recipe on page 126.

SWAP 2 PERCENT FOR FAT-FREE MILK.

This Simple Swap provides the same amount of calcium, but you'll save 39 calories per 8-ounce serving. And don't forget that a fat-free latte is a great way to kick up your calcium for the day! A "tall" size contains 8 ounces of milk, or 30 percent of your day's calcium requirement.

SWAP CHIPS FOR POPCORN.

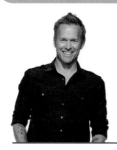

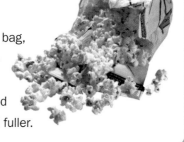

Even *baked* tortilla chips have 110 calories in a 1-ounce bag, and that's equivalent to less than 2 cups of chips. One ounce of air-popped corn (no butter!) has the same number of calories but more volume, yielding 4 cups (and providing 5 grams of fiber), so you can eat more and feel fuller.

Trainer Tip: BOB HARPER

Olive oil is not empty calories—it's good for you. It may be high in calories, but in moderation, it's a heart-healthy option.

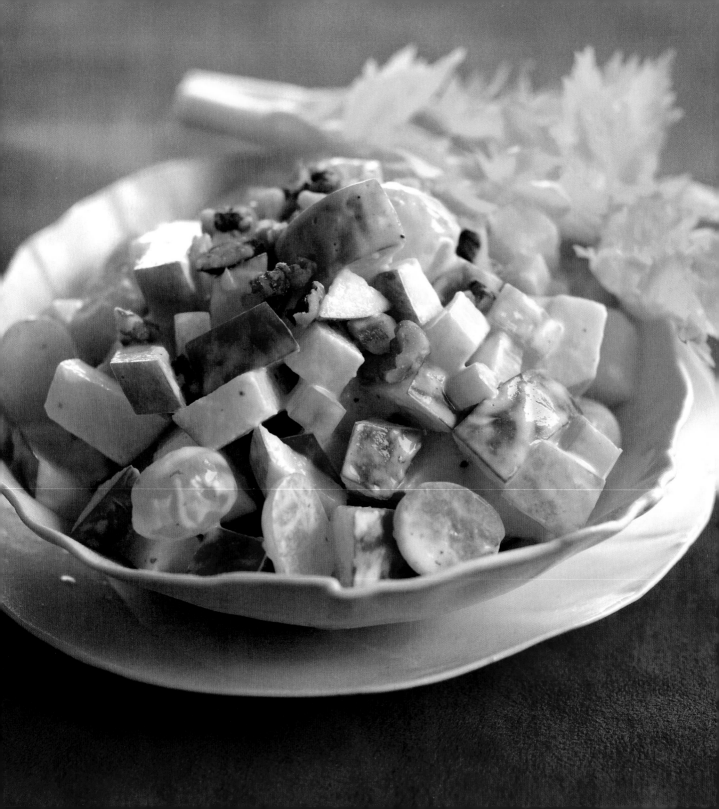

NUTTY WALDORF SALAD

The original Waldorf salad was invented by chefs at the Waldorf Hotel in New York City. The classic version was made with diced red-skinned apples, celery, and mayonnaise. My healthy reinterpretation is just as delicious, has fewer calories, and swaps bad fats for good.

2 medium apples (with peel), cored and cut in ½" pieces (about 2 cups)

½ cup chopped celery

½ cup sliced green grapes

6 tablespoons plain, fat-free Greek-style yogurt

1 teaspoon Dijon mustard

½ teaspoon lemon peel

¼ teaspoon salt

¼ teaspoon lemon juice

¼ teaspoon ground black pepper

2 tablespoons toasted chopped walnuts (see note)

In a mixing bowl, combine the apples, celery, grapes, yogurt, mustard, lemon peel, salt, juice, and pepper. Sprinkle with nuts just before serving.

Note: To toast nuts in the oven, preheat the oven to 375°F. Place the nuts in a single layer on a baking sheet and bake for 5 to 8 minutes, or until fragrant. Stir the nuts a few times during baking to ensure even browning. To toast on the stovetop, place the nuts in a small skillet over medium heat. Toast, stirring occasionally, for about 2 minutes, or until fragrant and lightly browned. Set aside to cool.

Makes 4 (³/₄-cup) servings

Per serving: 90 calories, 3 g protein, 16 g carbohydrates, 2 g fat (0 g saturated), 0 mg cholesterol, 2 g fiber, 200 mg sodium

Mo DeWalt, Season 8

One of the most important things for me to do once I leave the ranch is to be sure I eat out at places that prepare food in a healthy way, so that when I go out for a meal, I still eat like I did on the ranch.

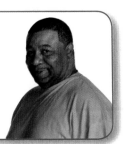

SWAP SUGAR FOR SWEET SPICES.

It's a good idea to start eating sugar-free yogurt and cereals, but you may miss the flavor of your old favorites. Try adding sweet spices such as cinnamon, nutmeg, and cloves to your favorite smoothies, cereal, yogurt, and even coffee or tea drinks. Not only do they add a delicious, sweet-spicy flavor, but they also contain antioxidants. Try stirring in a sprinkle of the pumpkin pie spice blend on page 114.

SWAP CANDY FOR SUGAR-FREE GUM.

If you like to chew something sweet, put down the toffees and pick up a pack of sugar-free gum. There are tons of flavors available, from mint to bubble gum. Chewing gum is also a great strategy to employ when you're distracted by thoughts of food but aren't actually hungry—it will keep your mouth occupied.

SWAP WHITE CRUMBS FOR WHEAT CRUMBS.

Don't forget that every crumb counts! Packaged bread crumbs and croutons are now available in whole grain varieties. Whether you're topping a salad or a healthy casserole, swap out the white stuff and you'll be rewarded with more crunch and hearty texture.

junk; and the heavy, greasy fast foods that they once ate without hesitation? Not an option anymore.

Sione Fa of Season 7 remembers that he used to eat two burritos a day—before lunch. "I was already way over my calorie intake for the whole day by noon," he says. "Then I would stop for lunch and have maybe three double cheeseburgers and a large order of fries. On the way home from work—my wife's going to kill me when she hears this—I'd grab the same exact thing and *then* eat dinner." But things have changed since he returned home from *The Biggest Loser* ranch. "Now I make sure that if I'm going to be away from home longer than 4 hours, I bring a healthy snack along with me so I'm not tempted by roadside food."

But it's not always easy to part with our favorite comfort foods—we've practically become addicted to empty carbs and refined sugar (not to mention salt!). The Simple Swaps and delicious recipes in this chapter will help ease you into this "white stuff" purge—you'll still satisfy your cravings without sacrificing your health or your weight-loss efforts.

When Season 7 winner Helen Phillips went home the first time after being on the ranch for several weeks, she found herself back in her favorite grocery store, smelling the pastries and doughnuts. "I was so afraid that my hand would just reach out and go back to my old ways." But Helen slowed down her panicked thoughts and realized there was a rainbow of fruit and vegetables in front of her.

"Something just clicked," she said. "I told my husband, 'I'm going to make you a dinner that's going to be beautiful and healthy. It's going to knock your socks off.'

"When I realized I was making the right choices, it was like, I get this. I have it. I can do it."

Eat to Keep Your Blood Sugar Steady

Foods like snack cakes, cookies, white pasta, chips, and soft drinks are all high in calories but very low in nutrition. They affect your blood sugar and insulin too quickly. And unlike their whole grain counterparts, these foods lack antioxidants and fiber, which are good for your digestion and can help prevent some types of cancer. In fact, these foods don't offer much of anything, other than calories. And remember, the quality of your calories is as important as the quantity.

Like many other overweight Americans, many *Biggest Loser* contestants arrive at the ranch each season with a diagnosis of type 2 diabetes—and the various pills and medications that go with it. They quickly learn the importance of keeping their blood sugar and insulin levels steady rather than letting them soar, then plummet, throughout the day.

And often after the contestants leave the ranch, their medications are no longer necessary. Fifty-four-year-old Ron Morelli of Season 7 found that his diabetes symptoms disappeared, as they did for his castmate, at-home grand prize winner Jerry Hayes, 63. Many other contestants who come to the ranch with prediabetes learn that they are no longer classified as having it after weeks of healthy eating and exercising.

Grocery Store Tour

Cranberries

Fresh cranberries are typically available in the fall and winter. Notoriously sour because of their high level of acid and very low sugar content, they're loaded with vitamin C. You can also buy them frozen, canned, or dried. Canned cranberries may contain added sugar, so when fresh ones aren't available, frozen berries are your best option. Dried cranberries are also a great addition to trail mix or cereal. When purchasing dried cranberries, be sure to choose those that are sweetened with fruit juice rather than sugar. Try the Cranberry Ginger Sorbet recipe on page 150.

Carbohydrates

Most of your carbohydrates each day should come from vegetables, fruits, and complex carbs, such as whole grain cereal (oats, bulgur), whole grain tortillas, brown rice, wild rice, and whole grain couscous. Your best strategy is to spread out your carb calories throughout the day rather than having a large bowl of cereal for breakfast or several slices of bread with dinner. This will prevent your blood sugar from spiking and crashing.

White flour, white sugar, white pasta, white bread, and processed baked goods affect your blood sugar and insulin too quickly—you don't want an excess of either in your bloodstream. And unlike their whole grain counterparts, these foods also lack antioxidants and fiber. Swap empty white carbs for nutritious foods that keep you feeling fuller, longer.

Sweeteners

When you add sugar to foods, you gain a burst of sweetness . . . and calories. But that's it—sugar doesn't contain any nutritional benefits; it is the definition of an empty calorie. Plus, sugar rapidly affects your blood sugar and insulin, causing it to spike, then drop—making you hungry, even if you've just eaten. The goal is always to keep your blood sugar on an even keel.

Among the contestants on *The Biggest Loser*, sweetaholics are legion. Ice cream, for example, came up several times as the "absolute favorite" food of several Season 8 contestants. But they learn to make substitutions, retrain their tastebuds, and eschew the roller-coaster ride of soaring and plummeting blood sugar. One of them, Abby Rike, says "My favorite, favorite food was chocolate ice cream, but I've learned to love frozen fruit mixed with *The Biggest Loser* Protein Powder and almond milk. It's a thick, creamy, delicious treat!"

Artificial sweeteners have become popular alternatives to white sugar, and there are countless varieties to choose from. For some people (including those with diabetes), artificial sweeteners are an integral part of their weight-loss efforts.

If you prefer not to eat artificial sweeteners, there are some natural alternatives to white sugar. Most of these options are not calorie free, but many offer health benefits, such as antioxidants,

Nutritionist Tip

For an easy, portable snack with a low glycemic load and only about 100 calories, choose an apple. Apples contain valuable vitamins, fiber, and pectin, which helps your body eliminate cholesterol. Apples also promote stable blood glucose levels while keeping you feeling full.

which are not found in sugar or artificial ingredients. As always, with these natural sweeteners, moderation is key. Below is a list of some natural sweeteners that contain nutrients and have low glycemic loads.

Agave nectar is extracted from the pineapple-shaped wild agave plant. It's a bit thinner in texture than honey, has a lighter taste, and contains antioxidants. Use sparingly, as 1 teaspoon has 15 calories.

Honey contains antioxidants, and dark-colored honey has the highest concentration. Eating local honey (harvested in your area) is also thought to help prevent seasonal allergies. Use sparingly, as 1 teaspoon has 21 calories.

Molasses is the dark-colored syrup that remains after some of the sugar has crystallized from the cane's juices during sugarcane processing. As a result, molasses has a relatively low sugar content. Blackstrap molasses provides calcium, iron, magnesium, and potassium, as well as a rich supply of antioxidants. Use sparingly, as 1 teaspoon has 16 calories.

Stevia is a no-calorie herb that's native to Paraguay. Because it's 300 times sweeter than sugar, only a very small amount is needed to impart sweetness to your food. It can be found in most health-food stores and contains no calories. Stevia is a pantry staple at *The Biggest Loser* ranch.

Xylitol is a white powder that occurs naturally

SWAP SALTY SNACKS FOR HOMEMADE CHIPS.

Instead of snacking on processed carbohydrates like crackers and chips, try making your own chips with whole wheat pita bread. Cut a pita in half and cut each half into eight triangles. Spread the pieces on a baking sheet, spritz with a little olive oil, and season as desired with spices such as garlic powder or chili powder. Pop into an oven preheated to 375°F and bake for about 8 minutes, and voilà! Delicious, healthy homemade snacks. Or try the Chili Lime Tortilla Chips recipe on page 145.

SWAP OATMEAL PACKETS FOR QUICK OATS.

While instant oatmeal packets are convenient, many varieties contain lots of sugar and little fiber or protein. Try making your own on-the-go packet by scooping ½ cup of plain quick oats into a resealable bag and adding your favorite mix-ins—such as cinnamon, fresh blueberries, or a tablespoon of walnuts. You'll also save money, since a tub of quick oats typically contains many more servings than a box of instant packets.

SWAP CORNFLAKES FOR BRAN FLAKES.

Cornflakes may be low in calories, but they're also low in fiber and protein. If they're your breakfast staple, you're probably hungry again before lunch. Instead, opt for bran flakes, which typically contain twice as much fiber and protein. Top with sliced banana or strawberries to add even more nutrients, antioxidants, and fiber.

SWAP CHOCOLATE SYRUP FOR COCOA POWDER.

Chocolate syrup is fat free, but it's loaded with refined sugar and calories, and doesn't offer the antioxidant benefits of chocolate. The next time you want to add some chocolate flavor to frozen yogurt or milk, sprinkle on unsweetened cocoa powder. One tablespoon has just 12 calories but packs big chocolate flavor.

Suzanne Mendonca, Season 2

For a sweet treat, I like to spread a graham cracker with fat-free cream cheese. I usually put fruit spread or fresh berries on top of it.

in many fruits and vegetables and is even produced by the human body during normal metabolism. It is made commercially from hardwood trees and fibrous vegetation such as birch tree bark or corncobs. Xylitol has the same sweetness and bulk as sugar but one-third fewer calories. Xylitol is also on hand in the ranch kitchen. Use sparingly, as 1 teaspoon has 10 calories.

Swapping White for Whole Grain

Unlike "white stuff," whole grain flours contain the nutritious bran and germ, as well as the endosperm, of the grain. The only downside to nutritious whole grains is that the bran and germ contain natural oils that can cause the flours to spoil more quickly than their highly processed counterparts. If you're not going to use whole grain flours immediately, it's best to refrigerate or freeze them for optimal shelf life.

High-fiber Ezekiel bread, a ranch staple, becomes a quick favorite of the contestants. Among the latest crop of cast members, Shay Sorrells says she's learned to replace potato hash at breakfast with Ezekiel raisin toast. And Sean Algaier says he's fallen in love with panini (Italian-style grilled sandwiches) made with 5 ounces of turkey, a slice of low-fat cheese, and two pieces of Ezekiel toast that have been grilled. "I *love* them!" he says with the enthusiasm with which he used to greet his

Grocery Store Tour

Raspberries

I never tire of raspberries for dessert. One cup has only 64 calories and a whopping 8 grams of fiber. Fresh raspberries can be expensive when not in season, but frozen raspberries are available year round and are typically more affordable. Keep frozen berries on hand for last-minute smoothies or to thaw and stir into yogurt or hot whole grain cereal.

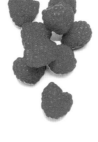

Watermelon

Watermelon is a ranch favorite. Besides the fact that everyone seems to love its flavor, watermelon is very high in water and quite low in calories. One cup contains 20 percent of your recommended daily vitamin C and only 45 calories. The lovely blush of color tells us it's also loaded with lycopene, a powerful plant chemical that helps prevent some types of cancer.

Grapes

Grapes make a refreshing cold snack, but they're also delicious halved or sliced and stirred into a salad. (Try the Nutty Waldorf Salad recipe on page 133.) Because they're harvested when ripe, they don't have a long shelf life, so buy just what you need, when you need them. Frozen grapes also make a refreshing treat at only 60 calories per cup. And when they're frosty, you're also likely to eat them more slowly!

Cocoa Powder

Loaded with antioxidants and very low in calories, just 1 tablespoon of cocoa powder can add a lot of rich flavor to a healthy concoction such as the Raspberry Smoothie on page 171. When purchasing cocoa powder, look for the natural, not Dutch-process, variety. Natural cocoa powder contains more antioxidants. You can find cocoa powder in the baking aisle.

daily three or four drive-thru cheeseburgers.

Though there are multiple types of whole grain flours available (amaranth, barley, cornmeal, oats, quinoa, rice), when it comes to baking at home, opt for wheat flour. Whole wheat flour contains the most gluten, a protein that gives baked goods structure, integrity, and the ability to rise, or leaven. To incorporate other whole grain flours into a recipe, you can replace one-quarter to one-third of the wheat flour with another type of flour. This will allow you to add a variety of nutrients, flavors, and textures without sabotaging your baking.

Today, a wide variety of whole grain products can be found in most grocery stores. Look for pasta and cereals, breads, tortillas, and crackers that list "whole wheat" or a whole grain as the first ingredient on the label. Be careful with products whose labels say "multigrain." They sound healthy, and they may indeed contain multiple grains. They may not be *whole* grains, however.

Mike Morelli, Season 7

I'm a different person now. My favorite meal used to be really anything from a drive-thru. On the way home, I used to stop at a fast-food place and get a couple of cheeseburgers, about 1,000 calories. It was closet eating at its worst. I'm not that person anymore.

SWAP MILK CHOCOLATE FOR DARK CHOCOLATE.

Chocolate is chocolate—there's no substitute for it! But a Simple Swap can make your next chocolate choice *better*. Rather than eating a milk chocolate bar, opt for a small piece of dark chocolate, which contains powerful antioxidants and may help to lower blood pressure. The flavor is rich and intense, so a small piece goes a long way. Look for chocolate that contains at least 60 percent to 70 percent cocoa solids. Cocoa nibs, which are bits of roasted cocoa beans, are also a good choice though they are often more expensive.

CHILI LIME TORTILLA CHIPS

I used to buy fried tortilla chips that were seasoned with chili and lime. They were absolutely addictive. My local grocery store seems to have stopped carrying them, so I've been forced to invent my own version. I think these are just as delicious and they are much lighter in fat and calories.

12 (6") corn tortillas

2 teaspoons chili powder

2 teaspoons True Lime powder (see note)

Salt, to taste (optional)

Preheat the oven to 300°F. Stack the tortillas and cut into eighths to make chips. Transfer to a baking sheet.

In a small bowl, combine the chili powder, True Lime powder, and salt (if desired). Mist the chips lightly with olive oil cooking spray and toss with the seasonings. Spread out the chips in a single layer on two large baking sheets.

Bake for 30 to 35 minutes, or until light golden and crisp, rotating the baking sheets once about halfway through. The chips will get crisper as they cool.

Makes 12 (8-chip) servings

Note: To find True Lime powder in a store near you, go to www.truelemon.com. True Lime is typically found in the baking aisle with the artificial sweeteners.

Per serving: 70 calories, 2 g protein, 12 g carbohydrates, 1 g fat (0 g saturated), 0 mg cholesterol, 2 g fiber, 50 mg sodium

Sean Algaier, Season 8

My tastes have changed a lot. I don't crave sugar like I used to, and I can say no to fast food. It's weird to think I would ever love or crave good-for-me food, but it's true!

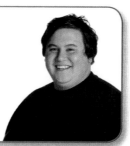

JERRY AND ESTELLA'S CHERRY CRUNCH

This recipe is a routine Simple Swap that Jerry and Estella Hayes of Season 7 created to replace their old after-dinner ice cream routine. Simple, crunchy, and sweet, it's their favorite choice for those nights when they have enough calories left in their daily budget for a sweet indulgence.

1 cup frozen or fresh sweet cherries, pitted

¾ cup fat-free Greek-style yogurt

2 teaspoons (2 packets) Truvia Natural Sweetener or other natural sweetener

½ cup Kashi GoLean Crunch cereal

Heat the frozen cherries in the microwave in a microwave-safe container for about 30 seconds. Combine the yogurt and sweetener. In a parfait glass, layer the yogurt and cherries and top with the cereal. Serve immediately.

Makes 2 (¾-cup) servings

Per serving: 130 calories, 11 g protein, 23 g carbohydrates, 1 g fat (0 g saturated), 0 mg cholesterol, 4 g fiber, 80 mg sodium

Nutritionist Tip

Fruits and vegetables occupy a lot of space in your stomach because they're high in water and fiber, but they're low in calories. Not only are they packed with vitamins and antiaging chemicals, but they make you feel full!

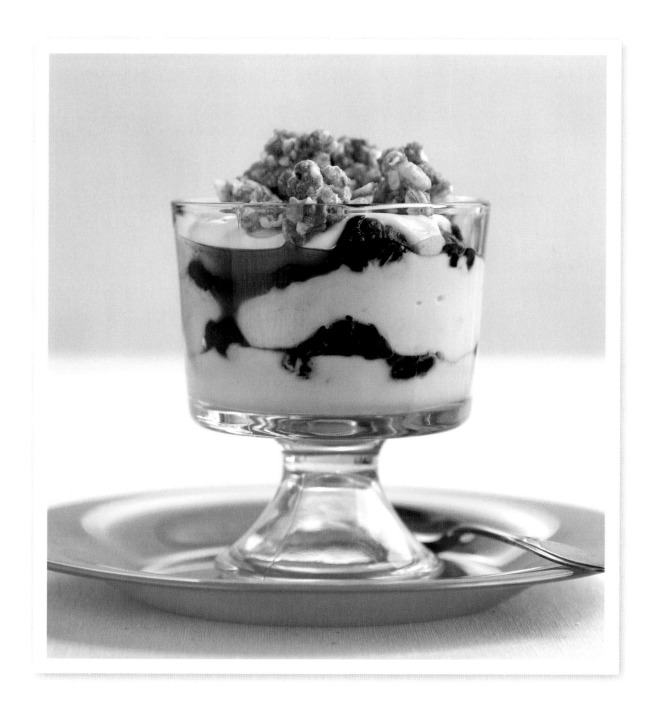

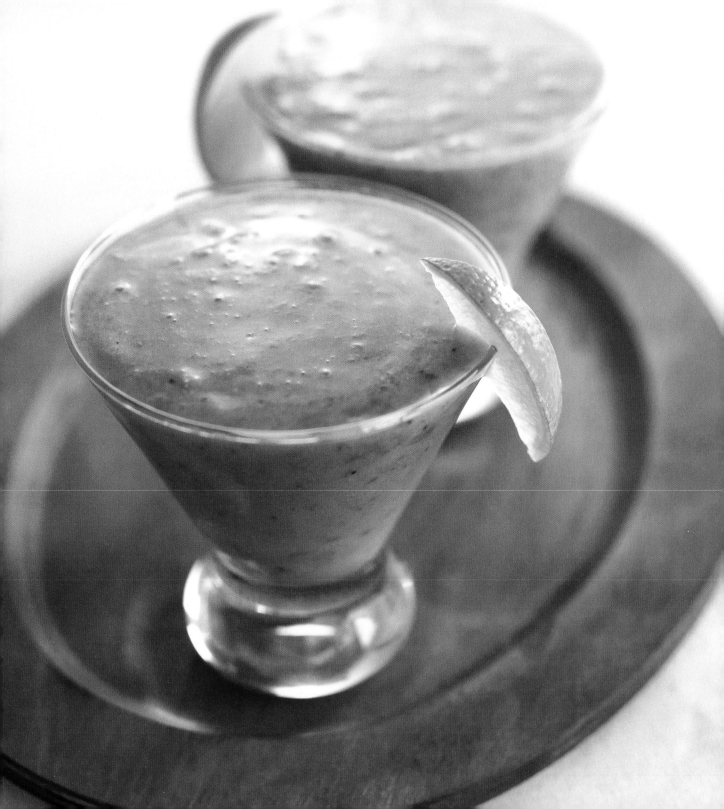

DANIEL'S FROZEN STRAWBERRY PARFAIT

Daniel Wright, who has spent two seasons at The Biggest Loser *ranch, likes to make this refreshing, invigorating snack after his morning workout.*

⅔ cup frozen or fresh unsweetened strawberries or other fruit

¼ cup (2 ounces) unsweetened vanilla Almond Breeze nondairy beverage

1 teaspoon (1 packet) Truvia, xylitol, or other natural sweetener

Combine the strawberries, Almond Breeze, and sweetener in a blender and blend, repeatedly pushing the frozen fruit to the bottom to ensure that the mixture is smooth and well blended. Serve immediately.

Makes 1 serving

Per serving: 45 calories, 1 g protein, 10 g carbohydrates, 1 g fat (0 g saturated), 0 mg cholesterol, 2 g fiber, 45 mg sodium

Antoine Dove, Season 8

Be careful when you drink calories. If you drink a bottle of soda, that can be hundreds of calories. One large strawberry is about 5 calories. When you think about it like that, that's where the strategic part comes in. You can eat a lot of healthy stuff that's filling and lower in calories.

MINI APPLE GINGERBREAD CUPCAKES

These irresistible little cakes are spicy but not too sweet. For sweeter flavor, you can add an additional tablespoon of your favorite sweetener to the batter.

2 cups stone-ground whole wheat flour

1 teaspoon baking soda

¼ teaspoon salt

2 teaspoons ground ginger

1 teaspoon ground cinnamon

¼ teaspoon ground cloves

¼ teaspoon ground nutmeg

⅔ cup low-fat buttermilk

½ cup molasses

⅓ cup canola oil

1 large egg

1 large egg white

1 teaspoon pure vanilla extract

1 cup finely chopped apple (sweet apple such as Fuji or Delicious, not Granny Smith)

Preheat the oven to 350°F. Lightly coat 30 mini-muffin cups with cooking spray. Set aside.

In a medium mixing bowl, combine the flour, baking soda, salt, ginger, cinnamon, cloves, and nutmeg. Set aside.

In another bowl, whisk together the buttermilk, molasses, oil, egg, egg white, and vanilla extract. Make a well in the dry ingredients and pour in the liquid mixture. Stir until just combined.

There will be about 3 cups of batter. Divide the batter between the prepared muffin pans.

Bake on the center rack for about 15 minutes, or until a toothpick inserted in a muffin comes out clean. Cool for about 10 minutes before removing from the pans.

Makes 30 mini-muffins

Per serving: 70 calories, 1 g protein, 10 g carbohydrates, 2 g fat (0 g saturated), 0 mg cholesterol, 1 g fiber, 90 mg sodium

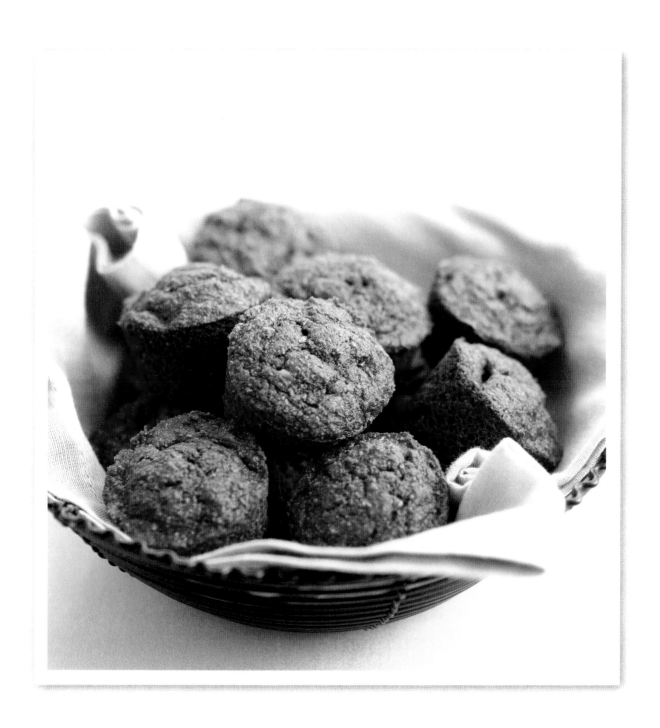

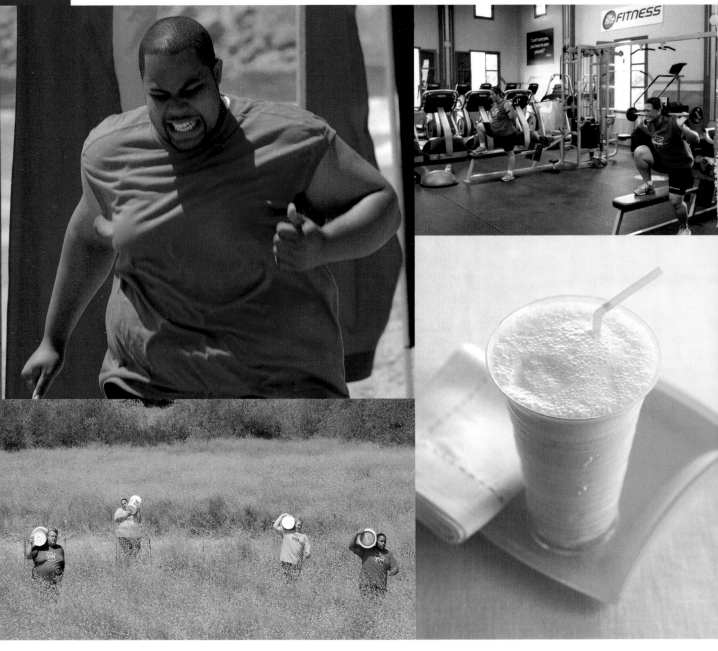

9

Eat, Don't Drink, Your Calories

Where there are burgers and fries . . . there's soda. As we've now firmly established, fast-food burgers were a major fixation for most *Biggest Loser* contestants before they arrived at the ranch. So it's no surprise that soda was a major source of calories, as well.

It's astounding how much soda (including diet) plays a role in the lives of many contestants. And if it's not soda, it's sweet juices and sports drinks or latte this or mocha that, every one of them chock-full of the same thing: empty calories.

Tom Desrochers Jr. of Season 6 used to rack up three 32-ounce containers of sports drinks a day, plus a few cups of regular soda. Add to that several cups of apple juice a week and we're talking a serious number of calories. His teammate and dad, Tom Desrochers Sr., didn't fare much better. His breakfast of pickles was accompanied by diet soda, and he professed a hatred of water.

Season 5 winner Ali Vincent was a breakfast latte girl, partial to the kind with whipped cream and caramel and all the trimmings. As she found out at the ranch,

Trainer Tip: JILLIAN MICHAELS

One simple step you can take at home to help you stay healthy is drinking water. It increases metabolism, helps muscle tone, and reenergizes you after exercise. It's hard to lose weight if you're not drinking enough water.

breakfast should not be an opportunity for dessert, and starting her morning with something sweet just set her up for wanting more sweet calories throughout the day. She still enjoys her steaming hot lattes, but now the word *nonfat* comes out first when she places an order, and she holds the "whip."

In this chapter, you'll learn why drinking enough water is so important (trust us—it is!) for health and weight loss, the many benefits of fat-free milk, and Simple Swaps for getting more of the right liquids into your life. Remember, the goal is to actually *chew* your calories—not slurp them through a straw!

With the exception of milk, protein powder, and fresh smoothies, *The Biggest Loser* eating plan motto is **Eat your calories.** That may sound obvious, but you'd be surprised. When they arrive at the ranch, most contestants (like most Americans) have absolutely no idea how many calories they consume each day through beverages alone—before they've even accounted for a single bite of food.

Season 7's David Lee, like many southerners, loves his iced tea, especially when it's sweet. When he first arrived on campus and sat down for his nutritional consultation, we did the math on his daily calorie intake from beverages alone. The results (shown below) were shocking.

David's Total Daily Average Intake of Sweet Tea and Soft Drinks

4.5 sweet teas (653 calories total)
+ 7.5 20-ounce sodas (1,999 calories total)
= 2,652 calories

David's total daily calorie budget at the ranch was less than he used to consume in drinks alone.

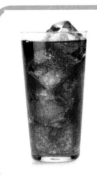

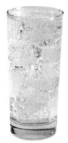

SWAP DIET SODA FOR FIZZY WATER.

Diet soda may be calorie free, but it often contains caffeine, sodium, artificial sweeteners, phosphoric acid, and other chemicals, and has even been linked to metabolic syndrome (a condition that can increase the risk of developing heart disease). If you really crave something bubbly, opt for sparkling water or seltzer instead.

Abby Rike, Season 8

I'm amazed at how easy the switch to better foods has been. I was addicted to diet soda. Six a day. Maybe I drank half a cup of water a day, and now I drink nothing *but* water. With all the healthy foods I'm eating, I'm full. I'm satisfied. . . . I'm shocked!

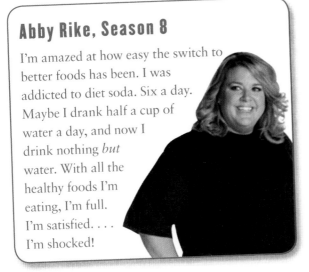

And it wasn't just the calories—with all of that soda and tea, he was taking in a whopping 1,019 milligrams of caffeine and 3½ cups of sugar, to boot. Talk about empty calories.

Water, Water Everywhere

If you're not already doing so, make sure you're drinking eight 8-ounce glasses of water a day to stay properly hydrated. This is especially important when you're changing your food habits and eating more fiber than your body is used to. Record your water intake each day in your food journal to be sure you've met your quota.

We tend to take water for granted, but it's something of a miracle elixir. Water provides a number

SWAP THE JUICE CARTON FOR A PITCHER.

Fruit juices are full of sugar and calories. Ditch the carton and invest in a water filter pitcher to keep cold, clean water in your fridge at all times. Aim to drink 2 quarts a day.

SWAP TONIC WATER FOR CLUB SODA.

Tonic water looks harmless, but one serving can contain more than 80 calories and 20 grams of carbohydrates! If you love your tonic water, try swapping it for calorie-free club soda or a sugar-free flavored sparkling water instead.

SWAP SPORTS DRINKS FOR PROTEIN SHAKES.

While you're working out, it's important to stay hydrated with water. But once your workout is over, don't pick up a sugary sports drink—opt for a protein shake, which will help your body rebuild muscle tissue more quickly. Try the Frosty Orange Protein Blast on page 166.

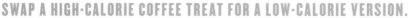

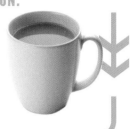

SWAP A HIGH-CALORIE COFFEE TREAT FOR A LOW-CALORIE VERSION.

Skip the sugary concoctions topped with whipped cream and syrup (some of which have more calories than a meal!) and order a small coffee or latte with skim milk, plus a sprinkle of cinnamon to add sweetness. You'll get the benefits of calcium and antioxidants without all the sugar and fat.

of benefits for overall health and weight loss in addition to proper hydration, which is essential if you're working out regularly. Staying hydrated improves all bodily functions at the cellular level and helps your heart and kidneys work more efficiently. In addition, water carries glucose, nutrients, and dietary antioxidants to our tissues, resulting in an energy boost and other health benefits. And water actually helps regulate body temperature (especially important for people with poor circulation) and increases satiety, or the feeling of fullness. In fact, some studies have shown that drinking a large glass of water 30 minutes before a meal can help reduce calorie intake during the meal.

And as trainer Bob Harper points out, when you're working out, it's important to drink water *before* you feel thirsty. "Chances are that if you notice you're thirsty," he says, "you've waited too long to drink, and your body is getting dehydrated. Keep water with you at all times when you're exercising."

When they arrive at the ranch, *Biggest Loser* contestants are immediately given their own refillable water bottles that they're rarely caught without. They constantly refill them throughout the day with filtered water that they guzzle as they sweat through their workouts and even when they rest. At any given moment, when a contestant is walking

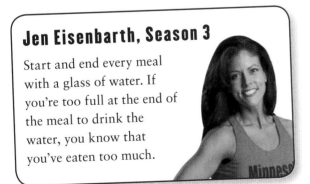

Jen Eisenbarth, Season 3

Start and end every meal with a glass of water. If you're too full at the end of the meal to drink the water, you know that you've eaten too much.

pound called epigallocatechin gallate (EGCG), which is a powerful antioxidant. Green tea is thought to have health benefits ranging from combating Alzheimer's disease to fighting some forms of cancer. In terms of weight loss, EGCG has been observed to have a mild metabolism-boosting effect.

While green tea does contain caffeine, the caffeine in green tea is surrounded by tannic acid compounds, which slow its release into the bloodstream. This effect, in addition to an overall lower caffeine level, results in fewer feelings of agitation or jitters than you sometimes get from coffee.

Black tea does not contain EGCG, because black tea leaves are oxidized during the fermentation process—but black tea still contains antioxidants and offers health benefits. Research suggests that black tea may help promote heart health by improving blood vessel function, and black tea is also thought to have cancer-fighting properties.

to the gym, tackling a challenge, or even simply being interviewed, that water bottle is present.

Tea Time

Hot or iced, unsweetened tea is a zero-calorie beverage that offers a lot of nutritional benefits. Green tea is an especially good choice, as it contains a com-

SWAP FRUIT JUICE FOR THE REAL THING.

Not only does a medium orange have half the calories of a 12-ounce glass of orange juice, but it also contains much more fiber, and it takes longer to eat than a glass of juice takes to drink. The sugars from whole fruits are released more slowly into your bloodstream than those from juice, so eating fruit prevents a hunger spike.

Common black tea blends include Earl Grey, English Breakfast, and Darjeeling.

Herbal teas are not really teas at all. These beverages, which are available in countless varieties, from chamomile to ginseng, are made from the roots, stems, flowers, seeds, and leaves of plants, not from tea leaves. They contain no caffeine and can be a good option when you're craving a calorie-free drink. Try ginger tea to calm an upset stomach or mint tea to decrease feelings of hunger.

Good to the Last Drop

Many of us can't bear to greet the day without a steaming cup of joe; just the smell of coffee brewing at the ranch is enough to motivate many contestants to get up for their morning workout. But this beloved brew does much more than jolt us awake on lazy mornings or deliver a welcome kick start when our energy is lagging.

Coffee contains natural antioxidants, which may protect against certain types of cancer (especially in women) and type 2 diabetes. Research has also shown an association between coffee consumption and decreased risk of Alzheimer's and Parkinson's diseases.

As we all know, coffee also contains caffeine, a phytochemical (plant chemical) that acts as a stimulant to the central nervous system. In moderation, caffeine can promote increased alertness and energy, though too much caffeine can result in anxiety, nervousness, and jitters.

Biggest Loser contestants find that cutting back on overall caffeine consumption, combined with getting exercise and eating nutritious foods, helps them get a better night's sleep—rest that they need for demanding workouts with Bob and Jillian!

Ever since caffeine was discovered in coffee some 200 years ago, curious scientists have been trying to find the best method of removing it. There are many

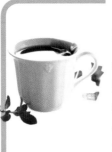

SWAP HERBAL TEA FOR GREEN TEA.

Antioxidant-rich green tea offers many health benefits—including lowered blood pressure, decreased cholesterol absorption, defense against cancer, and protection from tooth decay. It has also been reported that green tea can boost metabolism. In one study, people who drank 3 to 4 cups daily burned an additional 80 calories!

Grocery Store Tour

Milk

One cup of milk provides 30 percent of your recommended daily calcium. Swapping to lower-fat milks can be a challenge in the beginning, but at the ranch, most contestants adjust quickly when they see how many calories they can save. Personally, I like 1 percent milk in my coffee, so I keep both fat-free and 1 percent in my fridge. Here are the calorie breakdowns to give you some incentive to swap:

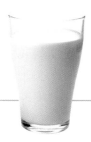

1 cup whole milk (3.25 percent fat) = 146 calories

1 cup 2 percent milk = 122 calories

1 cup 1 percent milk = 102 calories

1 cup fat-free milk = 83 calories

variables in making decaffeinated coffee, such as the type of bean used and the roasting and brewing techniques. As such, caffeine content in decaf coffee varies widely from cup to cup. The FDA states that decaffeinated coffee must have 97 percent of the caffeine removed from a green (unroasted) coffee bean. But since the average green coffee bean contains 1 to 2 percent caffeine, the amount of caffeine left in the bean can vary. Still, decaf can be a good option for people who have a serious coffee addiction and want to cut down on their caffeine intake.

Limiting Caffeine

The average American adult sips about 200 milligrams of caffeine a day, mostly from coffee (see the chart on page 162 for caffeine content of many popular beverages). Caffeine can have a number of adverse effects on your body. It can interfere with your sleep cycle, especially if you drink beverages with caffeine during the late afternoon and evening. And caffeine also causes a brief rise in the amount of calcium that escapes your body. Moderate caffeine consumption may not play a major role over the long term, but if you're not getting sufficient calcium in your diet, those small losses could add up to significant bone loss. Some studies have indicated lower bone mineral density or faster bone loss in postmenopausal women who drank 2 or more cups of coffee daily and got enough calcium. So if you drink even a moderate amount of caffeine, make sure you're getting plenty of calcium to protect your bones.

BEVERAGE OR OTHER PRODUCT	SERVING SIZE	CAFFEINE CONTENT (MCG)
Coffee, brewed	8 ounces	137
Black tea, brewed	8 ounces	65
Iced tea, black, instant	8 ounces	47
Espresso	2 ounces	42
Dark chocolate, bittersweet	1 ounce	20
Green tea, brewed	8 ounces	40
Natural unsweetened cocoa powder	1 tablespoon	12
Decaf green tea	8 ounces	5
Decaf coffee, brewed	8 ounces	2
Diet soda	12 ounces	46
Coca-Cola Classic	12 ounces	34

The Eat-Your-Calories Exception: Milk

Like most Americans, many *Biggest Loser* contestants simply weren't getting enough calcium in their diets. It's so important to keep your bones supplied with the calcium you need to stay strong.

During adulthood, you need 1,000 milligrams of calcium daily.

Trainer Jillian Michaels often encourages her contestants to drink a preworkout glass of fat-free milk to provide the fuel to keep going.

Weight-bearing exercise and resistance training are especially helpful for building bone strength. Weight-bearing exercises include dancing, jogging, jumping rope, and walking. The vibrations that go through your bones each time your feet strike the ground encourage better bone density. Resistance training is another form of bone-building exercise and includes lifting weights and using resistance bands as well as doing yoga and Pilates. Make sure to include these types

Nutritionist Tip

When a woman reaches age 50, her daily calcium need jumps to 1,200 milligrams. Women 50 and over may want to choose at least two servings of low-fat dairy per day to keep their bones strong and help prevent osteoporosis.

of exercise in your regular fitness routine.

If you're following *The Biggest Loser* food plan, you should be meeting your daily calcium needs. The traditional sources of calcium in the American diet are dairy foods, and consuming fat-free or low-fat milk, cheese, and yogurt will help you meet your needs. But nondairy foods such as leafy green vegetables, and canned wild salmon and sardines that contain edible bones, are also great sources of calcium. In addition, fruits and vegetables contain vitamins and minerals that help you absorb the calcium you get from your diet. And making Simple Swaps—such as replacing the water in your oatmeal with milk or swapping your usual salad greens for kale, spinach, or collard greens—is an easy way to include more calcium in your diet without blowing your calorie budget.

SWAP WINE FOR A SPRITZER.

We all know that alcohol has a lot of calories, so it's best to avoid it when you're trying to lose weight. But if it's a special occasion and you want a treat, order a white wine spritzer, which is a mix of half wine and half seltzer. It has half the calories (and alcohol) of a glass of wine and won't blow your calorie budget.

SWAP SWEET TEA FOR SUN TEA.

Not all iced tea is unhealthy—but when you pour in the sugar, it sure is! Iced tea that comes in cans, bottles, and mixes is loaded with sugar and artificial flavorings. Brew your own tea at home by placing four to six tea bags in a 2-quart glass container and letting it brew in the sun for 3 to 5 hours. Pour over ice for a refreshing, calorie-free beverage. For extra flavor, you can also add fresh mint leaves or lemon slices.

Pete Thomas, Season 2

Stay hydrated with lots of water to keep your body burning fat. If you hit a plateau, it may be because you're dehydrated.

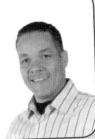

POMEGRANATE SPRITZER

This tasty and festive drink is easy enough to make any day of the week and pretty enough to serve to guests for a special occasion.

4 ounces lime-flavored sparkling water, chilled

2 ounces pomegranate juice, chilled

Fresh lime

Pour the sparkling water into a regular drinking glass or a festive champagne glass. Slowly add the pomegranate juice. Garnish with a slice of fresh lime.

Makes 1 serving

Per serving: 35 calories, 0 g protein, 9 g carbohydrates, 0 g fat (0 g saturated), 0 mg cholesterol, 0 g fiber, 10 mg sodium

SPICY ALMOND CHAI

The fragrance of masala chai is as intoxicating as its complex flavor. Chai is traditionally prepared by steeping spices in hot water and milk before adding black tea, but this rendition uses unsweetened almond milk and green tea instead. Delicious hot or cold, it takes just minutes to prepare.

4 cups water

6 (¼"-thick) slices peeled fresh ginger

½ teaspoon ground cardamom

1 (3") cinnamon stick

6 whole cloves

6 green tea bags

2 cups unsweetened almond milk

In a small saucepan over medium heat, combine the water, ginger, cardamom, cinnamon, and cloves. Bring to a boil, then reduce the heat and simmer for about 3 minutes. Remove from the heat. Steep the tea bags in the spice mixture for 5 minutes. Strain the mixture into a container and store for up to 1 week in the refrigerator.

To serve, combine the tea concentrate with the almond milk in a small saucepan. Simmer over low heat, but do not boil. Sweeten if desired. (To prepare a single cup, mix ⅔ cup hot tea concentrate with ⅓ cup hot almond milk.)

Makes 6 (1-cup) servings

Per serving: 15 calories, 0 g protein, 1 g carbohydrates, 1 g fat (0 g saturated), 0 mg cholesterol, 0 g fiber, 60 mg sodium

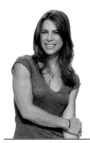

Trainer Tip: JILLIAN MICHAELS

Did you know that drinking one mocha latte a day adds up to an extra 42 pounds over the course of a year? So the next time you head over to your favorite coffee shop, try ordering a fat-free latte instead, or even better, try ordering a regular cup of coffee, which has zero calories.

FROSTY ORANGE PROTEIN BLAST

This creamy protein drink uses frozen orange juice concentrate to intensify the flavor without relying on additional sweeteners. It's a great postworkout snack.

2 cups unsweetened vanilla almond milk

1 (6-ounce) can frozen orange juice concentrate

1 cup plain, fat-free Greek-style yogurt

1 teaspoon pure vanilla extract

2 scoops (4 tablespoons) *The Biggest Loser* vanilla protein powder

16 ice cubes

Add the almond milk, juice concentrate, yogurt, vanilla, protein powder, and ice to a blender. Blend until smooth.

Leftovers can be poured into small zip-top bags and stored in the freezer. Thaw slightly and blend before serving.

Makes 4 (1¼-cup) servings

Per serving: 140 calories, 10 g protein, 23 g carbohydrates, 2 g fat (0 g saturated), 0 mg cholesterol, 4 g fiber, 135 mg sodium

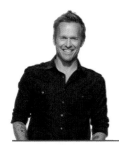

Trainer Tip: BOB HARPER

You need to make sure that after you've worked out, you give your body enough protein because you have to build the muscles back up after you've broken them down. Using *The Biggest Loser* Protein Powder is going to be helpful for you.

CARLA'S NO-CAL CITRUS COOLER

Carla Triplett of Season 7 never enjoyed drinking plain water, but when she added slices of lemon and lime, she liked the refreshing taste, and gradually she started adding even more fruit. Because this flavored water is virtually calorie free (eating the fruit will add up to a few extra calories), she can drink as much as she likes. This refreshing beverage is great after a tough workout.

1 lemon, sliced

1 lime, sliced

1 orange, sliced

10 red grapes

10 green grapes

4 cups water

Mint leaves

Wash the fruit thoroughly before slicing. Add the lemon, lime, orange, grapes, and water to a pitcher. Stir to mix the fruit. Refrigerate until chilled, then serve. Add mint leaves for added flavor.

Makes 4 (1-cup) servings

Per serving: 0 calories, 0 g protein, 0 g carbohydrates, 0 g fat (0 g saturated), 0 mg cholesterol, 0 g fiber, 0 mg sodium

Tom Desrochers Jr., Season 6

The harder you work out in the gym, the more water you need to drink to stay hydrated. More sweat doesn't just mean more weight lost; it also means you need to drink a lot more water. So always stay hydrated in the gym; it's key.

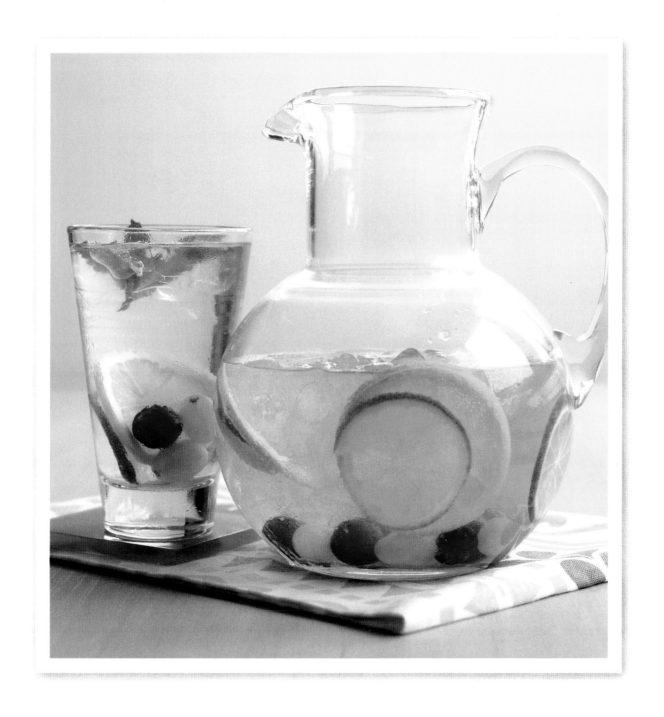

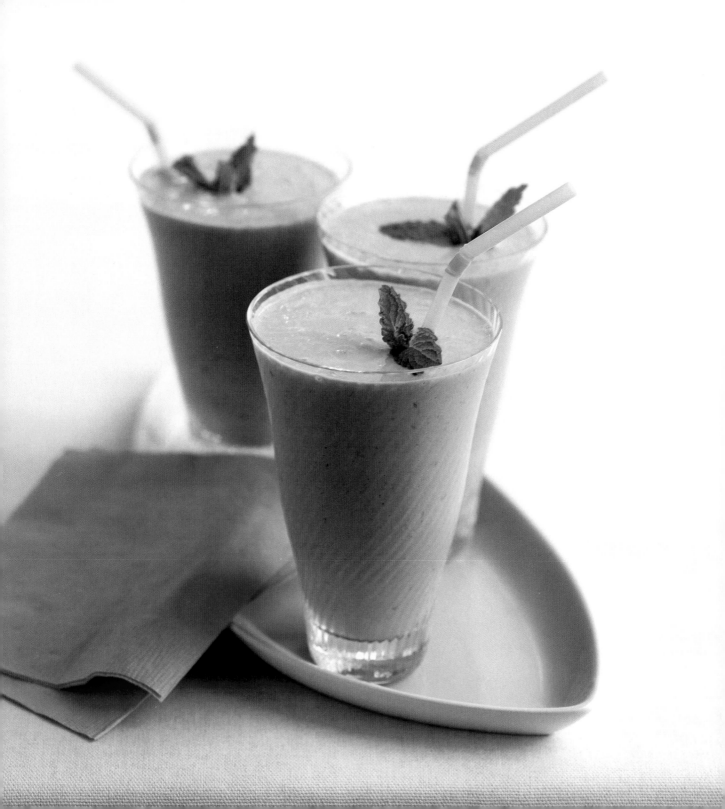

RASPBERRY SMOOTHIE

This is my idea of the perfect all-around snack. It takes minutes to make, satisfies a sweet tooth, and is high in both protein and fiber.

- 1 cup fresh or frozen raspberries
- ½ cup unsweetened vanilla almond milk
- 1 tablespoon unsweetened cocoa powder
- ½ cup fat-free Greek-style yogurt
- ½ teaspoon pure vanilla extract
- 1 packet stevia
- Ice cubes
- Fresh mint leaves

In the jar of a blender or the bowl of a food processor, combine the raspberries, almond milk, cocoa powder, yogurt, vanilla, stevia, and ice. Blend or process until smooth. Pour into glasses and serve immediately, garnished with mint.

Makes 1 serving

Per serving: 160 calories, 13 g protein, 21 g carbohydrates, 3 g fat (0 g saturated), 0 mg cholesterol, 10 g fiber, 125 mg sodium

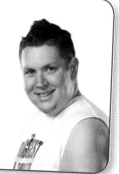

Neill Harmer, Season 5

Calories are like your daily allowance. Let's say you have 2,000 calories to spend per day. If you drink an iced latte with whipped cream and chocolate (400 calories), you just spent a *big* part of your allowance on something that really wasn't needed. Spend your calories wisely.

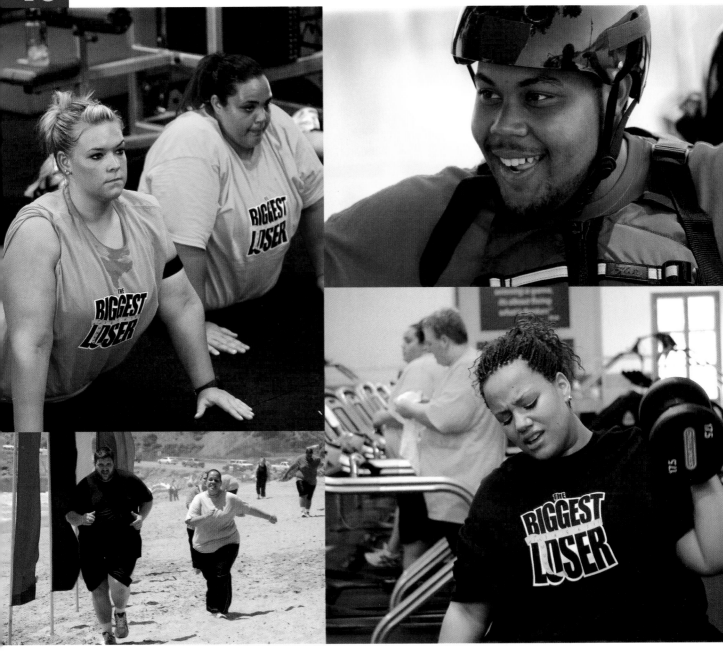

10

Moving Right Along

When the contestants arrive at the ranch, they're plunged immediately into fairly brutal workouts of 4 to 6 hours a day. There's no easing into the situation—they put down their suitcases and duffel bags, and *kaboom!* It's off to the gym with Bob and Jillian. A lot of sweat and tears (and maybe a little blood) are sacrificed in that gym, and when contestants emerge from their first workouts, they look a little like a herd of deer in headlights. In this case, however, they don't quite know what has already hit them.

No doubt about it, to lose weight, you have to burn more calories than you take in. And the best way to do that is to exercise. But now that you're learning to eat nutritious foods, prepare healthier meals, and make smarter choices, your body will be fueled and ready for more movement. Everyone starts out at a different level—from going for a 10-minute walk to running a 10-minute mile. Don't be afraid to start somewhere. Remember that the final four contestants of Season 7, much to their amazement, found themselves competing in a marathon by the last episode!

Trainer Tip: JILLIAN MICHAELS

For a fun workout, flip through a deck of cards and do the number of repetitions that corresponds to the number on the card. Face cards (such as jacks) equal 10 repetitions. An ace gives you a 1-minute break. Diamonds equal pushups, hearts equal lunges, spades equal crunches, and clubs equal reverse crunches. Keep going until you finish the entire deck.

No one expects you to run a marathon in a few months, and in fact, you should check with your doctor before you embark on any kind of exercise regimen. But you can turn your life around by degrees, and the best way to do that is through gradual change. Just swapping your old habits for ones that get you moving is a great place to start—ride your bike to work instead of driving, or get up and play with your kids in the park instead of watching them from a bench. No matter how you get moving, the end result is the same: weight loss, an increased energy level, and a brighter outlook on life.

Kristin Steede of Season 7, who dropped 132 pounds, said, "I used to be that person who would sit on the couch at home and watch the show. And I know how frustrated I was, seeing people on this show transform their lives forever. You sit at home and you want that so badly. I would just like to tell people that *it's inside of you, too.* You have it inside of you, and you just have to find it."

Stacey Capers, Season 6

If you work at a job where you sit most of the day, think about replacing your office chair with a stability ball. Or set an alarm on your computer or clock to remind you to get up and move— jog in place, walk up and down the stairs, or make the walk to the bathroom a brisk one.

Yes, You Can

At the ranch, contestants find out the hard way that they can do more with their bodies than they ever imagined possible. Fifty-something Bette-Sue Burklund of Season 5 used to sit in the gym with a

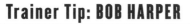

Trainer Tip: BOB HARPER

Most people don't know that taking the time to allow your body to recover is just as important as getting in cardio and weight training. Lifting weights is actually tearing down your muscle fibers, and it's only after the workout is finished that your body rebuilds that muscle. Also, never work out the same muscle groups on consecutive days. They need time to repair and recover.

10 Great Reasons to Stay Active

If you're like most people, you'll probably start exercising with one or two goals in mind: losing weight or toning up. But there are many more benefits. Here are 10 reasons to get moving and stay moving.

1. People who exercise live longer, on average, than people who don't.

2. Active people have a lower risk of dying of heart disease and stroke, and they're less likely to develop high blood pressure.

3. The more active you are, the lower your risk of colon cancer.

4. The less active you are, the higher your risk of developing type 2 diabetes. And if you already have type 2 diabetes, exercise can lower your blood sugar levels.

5. In people with arthritis, moderate exercise helps reduce joint swelling and pain and improves mobility.

6. Strength-building exercise helps counter bone loss (osteoporosis).

7. Exercise makes you "functionally fit," meaning that it becomes easier for you to carry groceries, do chores, and independently perform many other activities of daily life.

8. Because of the calming effect of exercise, active people are less depressed, and depressed people often feel better after they start exercising.

9. Exercise can save you money. If you can prevent serious—and costly—medical conditions such as heart disease, cancer, and osteoporosis, you'll have more money for your other needs.

10. Exercise can be fun! Many of the activities you did for play as a child count as exercise. Dancing fast, walking your dog, bicycling, and gardening all strengthen your heart and lungs.

towel draped over her head after a workout, convinced she was "going to die." Jillian had to lift up the towel and peer under to reassure Bette-Sue that she'd make it to the next workout.

It's human nature to listen to the negative voices in your head that tell you you can't do something. But it's crucial to get in the habit of overriding that negativity with positive energy. You have the power

SWAP SHORT-TERM THINKING FOR A LONG-TERM PLAN.

When you don't feel like going to the gym or you just don't think you can take another step on the treadmill, don't dwell on the moment: Focus on your long-term goals. Think of how good you'll feel when your workout is done, and how *great* you'll feel after you've lost the weight!

and the potential—you don't know how far you can go with exercise or anything else until you give it your all and go for it.

The trainers push the physical and mental limits of each contestant. The result? A stronger belief in themselves and their ability to do what they thought was impossible. It's that belief that fuels their motivation to get up day after day

and do the hard work necessary to lose weight.

In the end, the more you start moving and burning calories, the more you're going to love the way your body looks and feels—and that will be its own motivation. You'll be a new person inside and out.

How Much Is Enough?

The American Council on Exercise recommends 20 to 30 minutes of cardiovascular exercise 3 to 5 days a week, depending on intensity, and strength training at least twice a week. You can combine cardio and strength training on a given day or alternate the days you do each. For example, you might take a class at your gym that combines cardio and weights, or you might choose to ride your bike 1 day and do Pilates the next. Most former contestants typically strive for an hour to 2 hours 5 or 6 days a week to stay active and maintain their weight loss. And they always, *always* take at least 1 day of rest to allow their bodies to recuperate.

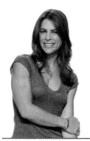

Trainer Tip: JILLIAN MICHAELS

If you already have a moderate level of fitness and you're looking to kick it up a notch, try adding some jump work to your routine. If you're doing squats, try a jump squat. Or try some jumping lunges. And for a little variety in your cardio, try jumping rope or doing jumping jacks.

Learn Some New Moves

- You don't have to be skinny to do yoga! There are lots of different levels of classes available to people of all skill levels. Or try it on your own with a video at home. Yoga helps you get in touch with and appreciate your body and what it can do—and it's a great workout.

- For more efficient fat burning, consider doing your cardio first thing in the morning—before breakfast. Your body is low on stored carbohydrates then and will more readily tap into fat for energy. A similar option is to perform your cardio workout after your circuit workout. Circuit training burns stored carbohydrates first; afterward, when you switch to cardio, your body calls on stored fat, since your carbohydrate reserve is depleted.

- Pool training is a great, low-impact way to burn calories that's easy on your joints. The trick is to keep moving in the water—swim laps, walk in the water, or tread water in the deep end. Use some pool toys, too, such as a flotation device that allows you to kick your way across the pool, or a pool buoy that you can place between your legs, letting them rest while you work your upper body. Working out in the pool is also a great option if you're injured.

Remember, **1 pound of body fat equals 3,500 calories.** By burning 250 to 500 calories a day through exercise, you could lose up to a whole pound a week (7 × 500 = 3,500), as long as you push yourself physically and stay within your calorie budget.

Exercise with a Smile

It's so important to find a physical activity that you actually enjoy doing. While they log their regular hours in the gym, many contestants also start

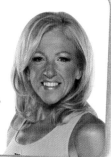

Helen Phillips, Season 7 Winner

You can do this at home. Take the 15 minutes you have, the half hour you have, and fit some sort of workout routine into it.

SWAP THE MINIBAR FOR A JUMP ROPE.

When you're traveling and find yourself alone in a hotel room, don't explore the minibar. Instead, take out the jump rope you packed in your suitcase and get some spontaneous exercise when boredom or downtime triggers an urge to snack. Try bringing your knees up high to increase the intensity (and calories burned!).

SWAP STANDING ON TWO FEET FOR STANDING ON ONE.

The next time you find yourself waiting in a line or having to stand in one place for a while, try lifting one foot off the floor. It'll help you work on your balance and strengthen your core muscles while you wait.

SWAP OLD SNEAKERS FOR NEW ONES.

If you've covered 350 to 500 miles in your sneakers or have had them from 3 to 6 months, it may be time to ditch them for a new pair. You're not doing yourself any favors by hanging on to the old ones—worn soles can cause painful foot problems such as plantar fasciitis, an inflammation of the tissue band (fascia) connecting the heel to the toes.

to participate in activities they really love, such as hiking (lots of mountains surround *The Biggest Loser* ranch), swimming, and yoga.

As they gain confidence in their strong new bodies, they also gain the confidence to experiment with new forms of physical activity. Cathy Skell of Season 7 began taking Spinning classes. Castmate Shanon Thomas joined her local roller derby when she returned home from the ranch. For Season 5 winner Ali Vincent, it was rediscovering her lost passion for swimming. Carla Triplett of Season 7 discovered she loved dancing in her own home. And Estella Hayes, also of Season 7 (and in her early sixties, we might add), discovered Zumba classes, a cardiovascular workout that blends salsa and hip-hop dance moves. Sampling different

Filipe Fa, Season 7

Put all doubt behind you and just work at it, because there's no greater feeling than accomplishing a solid workout every day. Every time I go into the gym, I remind myself of how good I'll feel afterward. Before, I used to walk into the gym— and walk back out.

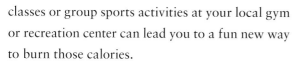

Shanon Thomas, Season 7

Find ways to keep moving. If you don't have time for the gym, go for a walk around your block or scrub your kitchen floor. You'd be surprised. Some days I burn 800 calories cleaning my house for an hour!

classes or group sports activities at your local gym or recreation center can lead you to a fun new way to burn those calories.

Signing up for a future athletic event is another way to make yourself commit to a daily training regimen. Participating in charitable events like walkathons or 5-Ks is a great way to exercise, meet people, and do some good in your community. In fact, many former *Biggest Loser* contestants reunite throughout the year at triathlons and

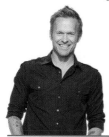

Trainer Tip: BOB HARPER

One of the biggest mistakes beginning runners make is to run too fast, causing shortness of breath and side cramps. To prevent this, concentrate on breathing deep down in your belly, and if you have to, take walking breaks.

SWAP DEFEAT FOR VICTORY.

So what if you missed your workout yesterday? Just get back to your workout plan today. Beating yourself up is not going to push you to your goal. It didn't work in the past, did it? There are no mistakes, just ways to learn.

SWAP SITTING AROUND FOR HELPING OTHERS.

Do you have an elderly neighbor or friend who could use some help around the house, mowing the lawn, planting a garden, raking leaves, or shoveling snow? Help them out and help yourself as well by being active on their behalf.

SWAP TIME FOR INTENSITY.

If you're short on time for your daily workout, try to make it more intense. If you're walking, look for an incline. If you're swimming, push a little harder. If you're at the gym, do reps a little faster. Make the most of the time you have by pushing yourself harder.

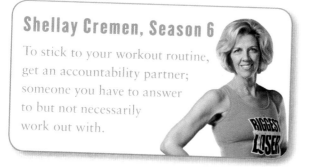

cise into your time there. Whether it's a cycling race in California, kayaking in Colorado, beach volleyball in Florida, or hiking the Appalachian Trail, get the whole family involved and make your time away from home more than an excuse to eat, drink, and sit on the beach.

Time for a Commercial Break

It's okay to watch some TV, but get creative about your time spent in front of the set. Don't just sit there during the commercial breaks (or worse, hit

other events across the country. Go online and look for upcoming events in your community or go to biggestloser.com and learn how you can lose weight and help feed America's hungry with the Pound for Pound Challenge.

Spending time away from home can also be a great way to inspire creative physical activity. While some vacations can undermine your weight-loss efforts, why not turn your next vacation into another reason to get fit? Think about where you'd like to visit and how you could incorporate exer-

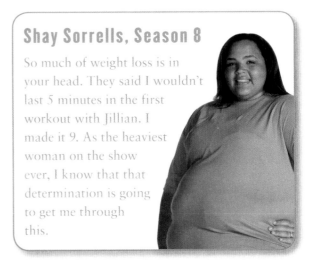

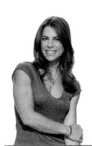

Trainer Tip: JILLIAN MICHAELS

To motivate yourself to exercise, think hard about your reasons for losing weight. Does it mean wearing skinny jeans? Having sex with the lights on? Playing with your kids for an hour? Get specific. Even better, write it down.

the fridge)—get up from the couch and do something active. You could do jumping jacks, lift free weights, knock out some pushups or crunches, take the dog out for a quick walk around the block, or climb up and down the stairs in your home. There are lots of possibilities—and those few extra minutes of activity can make a big difference. As Season 7's Blaine Cotter says, "The hardest workouts I do require just me and the floor. Everyone has a floor."

Also, start being mindful of how much TV you're really watching—it can add up to more than you might realize. Season 7 contestant Sione Fa admits, "My excuse for not working out used to be 'Oh, I don't have time.' But it was a lie. How was I able to get in 3 or 4 hours of TV every night if I didn't have time? There's time; you've just gotta

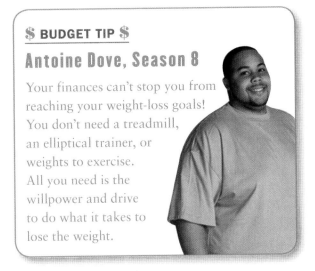

$ BUDGET TIP $

Antoine Dove, Season 8

Your finances can't stop you from reaching your weight-loss goals! You don't need a treadmill, an elliptical trainer, or weights to exercise. All you need is the willpower and drive to do what it takes to lose the weight.

SWAP EXCUSES FOR ACCOUNTABILITY.

Instead of turning off the alarm clock and sleeping in, or working overtime and not taking that walk you planned, recruit a workout buddy. You'll be less inclined to let yourself off the hook when you know someone is going to be showing up and looking for you.

SWAP YOUR DESK CHAIR FOR A STRETCH.

If you sit in a chair all day, take time to stand up for a stretch. Facing a wall from 3 feet away and with feet flat on the floor and knees locked, place your hands on the wall, lean forward, and hold for 10 seconds to allow your calf muscles to stretch. Repeat five times.

SWAP HIGH IMPACT FOR LOW IMPACT.

If your knees or joints are taking a pounding, focus on exercise that causes less stress to those areas, such as using an elliptical machine or recumbent bike, taking a Pilates class, or swimming. You can still get your heart rate up without aggravating any soreness or injuries.

make it." Not to mention, watching television and snacking go hand in hand—and as such, can be the ultimate enemy of weight loss.

All that television time can also have an impact on your family's health. In fact, not only has childhood obesity been linked to excessive TV viewing, but a recent study found that teens who watched more than 5 hours of TV a day were more likely to consume fast foods as adults. So put down that remote and get the whole family moving. Healthy habits start young!

Family is one of the biggest motivations for contestants at the ranch—it is often what inspired them to try out for the show, and what inspires them to keep going, even when they desperately miss life at home. "My kids deserve a healthier mom or dad" is a contestant quote heard over and over again. And family can also be what helps them stay active once they leave the ranch. Season

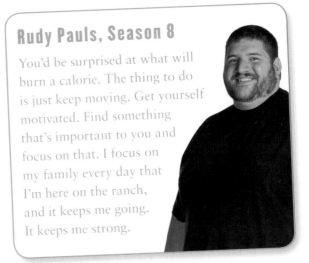

Rudy Pauls, Season 8

You'd be surprised at what will burn a calorie. The thing to do is just keep moving. Get yourself motivated. Find something that's important to you and focus on that. I focus on my family every day that I'm here on the ranch, and it keeps me going. It keeps me strong.

8's Allen Smith says he's already thinking about taking family walks with his wife and kids when he gets home.

The Great Outdoors

One of the best things about exercising outside is that it doesn't cost a thing—Mother Nature requires no membership dues. Getting out into the

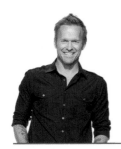

Trainer Tip: BOB HARPER

The hardest part of losing weight is often not having support. Find a friend, a family member, or even an online buddy to join you in your weight-loss journey. Studies show that having a partner increases weight-loss success. So buddy up and hit the gym.

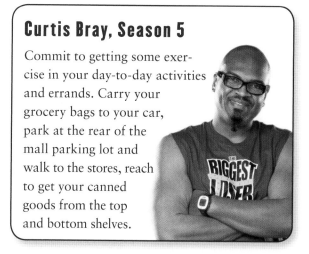

Curtis Bray, Season 5

Commit to getting some exercise in your day-to-day activities and errands. Carry your grocery bags to your car, park at the rear of the mall parking lot and walk to the stores, reach to get your canned goods from the top and bottom shelves.

fresh air also provides mental benefits. Abby Rike of Season 8 is incorporating a lot more walking and hiking into her new active life. She says, "Being outdoors is good for my mind, body, and soul." Amy and Phil Parham of Season 6 enjoyed their hikes at the ranch so much that when they got home, they made hiking with their sons a part of the family schedule.

Trainer Bob Harper is a big fan of outdoor activity and often takes his contestants outside for workouts that don't need any fancy equipment—just the use of their own body weight as resistance for squats, lunges, and all kinds of other heart-pumping exercises. Even if you belong to a gym and work out there most days, exercising outside

"can be a great way to break up the monotony of the gym," says Season 8's Danny Cahill.

Daniel Wright of Seasons 7 and 8 concurs. "I love the gym, but it can get old," he says. "On a nice day, ditch the gym and find a local park with trails. A good hike or walk can burn a lot of calories, and you'll love the view."

Exercising outdoors is also a great way to enjoy seasonal sports like ice skating, cross-country skiing, and snowshoeing. And some studies have indicated that exercising outdoors can have mental health benefits as well. British researchers found that people who exercised in an outdoor setting reported reduced levels of anxiety and depression compared to those who exercised indoors. So get outside and get moving!

Michelle Aguilar, Season 6 Winner

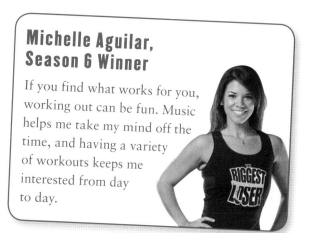

If you find what works for you, working out can be fun. Music helps me take my mind off the time, and having a variety of workouts keeps me interested from day to day.

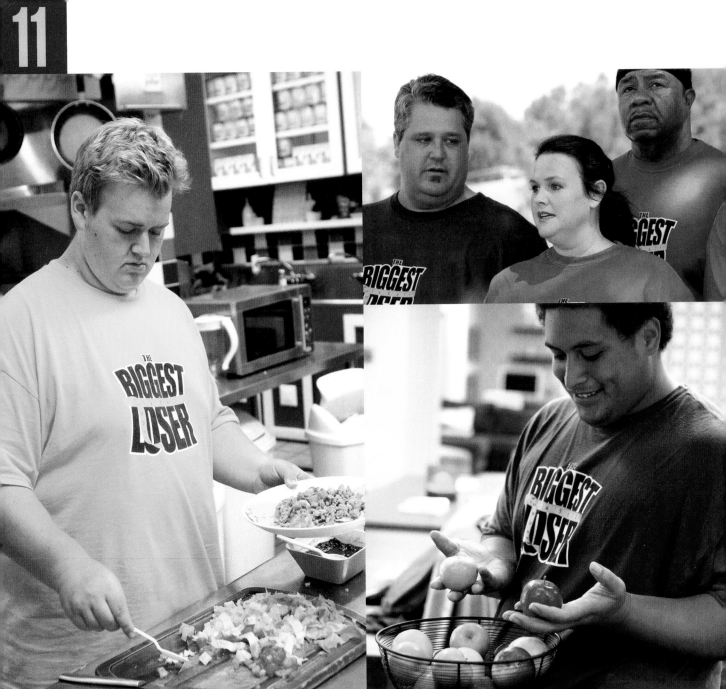

11

Creating a Game Plan for Life

Although *The Biggest Loser* contestants come to the ranch to lose weight and compete for cash prizes, at some point during their stay, they all realize that even more important than alliances, challenges, or money is the commitment they make to their health. Season 5 winner Ali Vincent says it took being eliminated, going home for several weeks, and then winning a place back at the ranch to realize how important it was to focus on the big picture. "I was glad to be back," she says. "I tried to convey to everyone that we're all going home eventually; our journeys are so much bigger than day-to-day ranch politics. I stopped obsessing about falling below the yellow line; I just focused on what I could control and did my best." Abby Rike of Season 8 understood what was at stake right away. "It's not a 3-month commitment," she said during her first week on the ranch. "It's not a 6-month commitment. It's a lifetime commitment. It never changes. For me, this isn't a game."

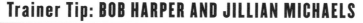

Trainer Tip: BOB HARPER AND JILLIAN MICHAELS

The journey our contestants take doesn't end once they leave the ranch. As many of you know, it can be hard to maintain healthy habits at home. That's why it's important to focus on small steps that sustain you. Try to include your friends in your workouts, cook healthy meals with your family instead of eating out, and focus on proper hydration.

SWAP VICTIMHOOD FOR EMPOWERMENT.

It's easy to fall into the pity trap, but feeling sorry for yourself and looking for others to blame for your troubles won't move you closer to your goals. Try to focus on what inspires you to make a change, and on the success you've had so far. See yourself as an example that will inspire and empower others to get healthy.

SWAP FEAR FOR COURAGE.

Practice doing one thing that scares you each day. If you're terrified of the gym, make yourself go for 10 minutes. If you're intimidated by cooking, ask a friend to join you and try making a healthy recipe together. Soon all the small steps will add up, and you will have made the leap into a healthy new lifestyle.

SWAP PERFECTIONISM FOR A HEALTHY BALANCE.

Nobody's perfect, and it's normal to experience mistakes and slipups when you make big changes to your life. Commit to making the best, healthiest choices you can 80 percent of the time. This leaves room for both planned and surprise indulgences, without sabotaging your weight-loss efforts.

Tara Costa, a Season 7 finalist, may not have won the grand prize but says that she did win her life back. "And that's even bigger," she says. "I'm done with life just passing me by. I want to start living again. I feel like I've changed inside and out, and it's the best experience I've ever had."

The ranch, the prizes, the trainers—it's all just icing on the cake. The true gift that *The Biggest Loser* gives the contestants is the power to change their lives. And that power comes from knowledge: understanding how their bodies work, why they've gained weight, the role of nutrition, and how to make healthy choices. You have in your hands that same knowledge, from the same experts the contestants rely on. The choice is yours. Today is the day to commit to a lifetime of health, to create a game plan for the future. It all starts with swapping your habits and making choices that support your long-term goals.

> ## Blaine Cotter, Season 7
>
> Why do you want to be healthy? I learned a valuable lesson on the ranch: The only way you're going to do the work and make lasting changes is if you love yourself enough to know that you're worth the effort.

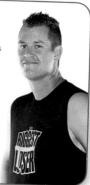

Dan Evans, Season 5

Listen for words of support when you're having a tough day. When I got home from the ranch, there were days I felt emotionally drained, and my body wasn't functioning at 100 percent. But my mom would say, "Dan, look how far you've come." I just needed to hear those words. It was like a little gust of wind in my sails to keep me going one more day.

The Ultimate Motivation

Moving forward, one of the most important components of your game plan will be motivation—you have to stay motivated if you want to achieve long-term success. For many *Biggest Loser* contestants, concern for their families is what motivates them to lose weight, and to keep going when things get tough. Whether it's a team of sisters, two cousins, or a parent coming to the ranch alone to create a better version of themselves for their kids back at home, all the contestants are aware that the state of their health and quality of life has a direct impact on their families.

A little past halfway through Season 7, contestant Kristin Steede realized that her time at the ranch was only the beginning of a much bigger journey. "This isn't about winning this game," she said. "This is about saving my life and hopefully saving the lives of other people who are in this situation. Win or lose, I plan on making an impact. I plan on helping people who are in the same situation as I was when I first got to the ranch, because I know how tough it is."

Dane Patterson, who lost 132 pounds in Season 7, says, "When I first arrived at the ranch, I was this 412-pound guy who felt he was letting his family down by not taking care of himself. I've rectified that."

Season 7's Sione Fa experienced a moment with his trainer that really sent the message home. "There was one thing Bob said to me: 'Be the man your family thinks you are.' To me, that's what I want to be. At this point in my life, it's losing weight. It's finding myself again so I can be the man they think I am."

And Aubrey Cheney of Season 7 says, "I can

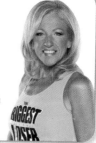

Helen Phillips, Season 7 Winner

If you keep a positive attitude and keep striving toward your goals, they can be attained. I'm living proof of that.

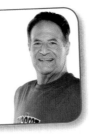

Ron Morelli, Season 7

It's not about winning a game show; it's about changing what's broken in your life.

now look back and realize how unhappy I was, how I was just going through the motions of life, but I wasn't living. I have had a taste now of what it's like to have energy and to be happy, to really mean the smile I put on my face. My kids are seeing a side of their mom that they haven't seen in a long time."

SWAP EMOTIONAL EATING FOR JOURNALING.

A journal is a safe place to share your feelings, fears, hopes, and dreams. Let out your emotions on paper, not in the kitchen, and listen to your inner voice instead of trying to comfort it with food. Journaling is an outlet you can turn to throughout your life, any day, any place. All you need is a pencil and paper.

SWAP SABOTAGE FOR SUPPORT.

If you feel that you're not getting the support you need from family and friends, it's crucial that you seek it out in other places, from sources you trust. Join an online weight-loss community such as BiggestLoserClub.com or look for a local weight-loss or athletic club that meets in your area. Spending time with like-minded people who support your goals and inspire you to keep going will increase your odds of success.

SWAP DEFEAT FOR SUCCESS.

Think of three tough challenges in your life that you overcame with resounding success. Then ask yourself what characteristics, strategies, and strengths helped you reach that success. Consider the obstacles you face now in light of this, and become aware of how you can rely on your strongest qualities to help pull you through again.

SWAP OTHER PEOPLE'S NEEDS FOR YOUR OWN.

This is one of the hardest changes for many *Biggest Loser* contestants to make, and why their time at the ranch—away from relatives, colleagues, friends, and others who place demands on their time—is so valuable. It's important to understand that putting your needs first is not selfish. Your health and happiness are more valuable than any PTA meeting or dinner party. Allow yourself to focus on *you*.

The Power of Commitment

Getting healthy is one thing. Staying healthy and maintaining weight loss is another. It requires a continued commitment to your health and continually reassessing your progress, and setting new goals. "Your mind can't stay the same," says Ron Morelli of Season 7. "It has to change along with your eating and exercise habits."

When he arrived at *The Biggest Loser* ranch, Ron weighed 430 pounds, and that was after having gastric bypass surgery several years earlier. He was the first postbypass contestant to appear on the show. Before undergoing the procedure, Ron weighed 527 pounds. "After the surgery," he says, "I got down to 340, then I climbed back up to 430 pounds over 13 years. My wife and I planned my funeral. I didn't think I would live a long life."

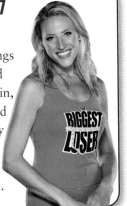

Tara Costa, Season 7 Finalist

For so long I didn't do things because of my weight. And now I've climbed a mountain, I've kayaked, I've competed in a marathon. . . . I finally feel like I'm alive and I'm doing things. This is my life now. I've taken it back.

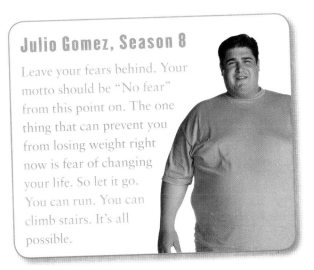

Julio Gomez, Season 8

Leave your fears behind. Your motto should be "No fear" from this point on. The one thing that can prevent you from losing weight right now is fear of changing your life. So let it go. You can run. You can climb stairs. It's all possible.

While gastric bypass surgery is successful for some people, it didn't work for Ron. Why? "I wasn't really committed to the notion that I had to change my lifestyle *after* surgery, that I had to eat right and exercise. Of course, if I could do that, I wouldn't have considered surgery. You've got to get the word *diet* out of your vocabulary," says Ron.

Developing a healthy lifestyle isn't about "dieting," and it's also not about short-term success. Fitting into your favorite jeans or losing 20 pounds for your high school reunion is a great achievement, but it's a short-term goal and should be celebrated as such. Your healthy living game plan must involve a commitment to your future goals.

What happens when you commit to a healthy lifestyle? Ron is an inspiring example. "I'm thinner than I've been in 40 years," he says. "I'm sitting

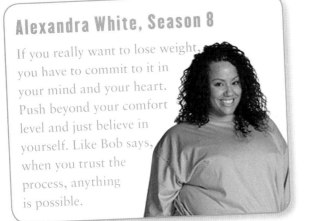

here with my legs crossed, which I haven't done forever. I'm not going back. I like this too much."

Digging Deep

Another important part of your game plan is allowing yourself to explore the feelings and emotions that are preventing you from moving forward. For Daniel Wright, a contestant in both Season 7 and Season 8, finding the motivation to keep up a healthy lifestyle meant really examining the issues that had gotten him where he was, before he could commit to a change that would take him where he wanted to go. "Examine yourself," he says. "Figure out the reasons for the weight gain. Look at stuff that is going on in your life. How you feel. Dig into that. Once you figure that out, you can begin to work on fixing that issue.

"I've got issues," he admits. "Those issues are why I ate my way to 450 pounds. For me, it was realizing that when I'm afraid of a tough situation, I run to food. More and more, I began to realize that I turn to food when I have problems, the same way other people turn to smoking or drinking. It was a crutch, a comfort, my source of joy in life. And what kind of life is that?"

Season 5 winner Ali Vincent says that losing weight for her was just as much an emotional transformation as it was a physical change. "Like a lot of people," she says, "when I felt hurt or confused or abandoned, I found solace in food. Eating was an emotional response to my problems, and it became a habitual response. I didn't know how to communicate and ask for what I wanted."

Ali says that process of losing weight and changing her priorities to fit her healthy new lifestyle forced her to grow up and let go of past hurts. "As I lost the weight, I gained maturity. As an adult, I can see situations and the actions of others for

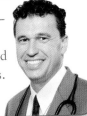

Dr. Jeff Levine, Season 2

Turn to relaxation techniques—such as tai chi, imagery, and deep breathing—instead of food when you want to reduce stress. They're calorie free!

what they really are. I understand that I'm not responsible for all the unpleasant things that happen in life. It's not about me."

Inspiration

The great thing about making healthy changes in your life is that you can have a positive impact on other people's lives as well. As you move forward with your game plan, think about who inspires you, and who you may be able to inspire by setting a positive example.

"I have an 8-year-old daughter," says Danny Cahill of Season 8. "She started getting a little chubby for her age at around 6 or 7 years old. One day she came into the living room and stuck her belly out and said, 'I've got a big belly like Daddy. I want to be just like Daddy.'" That was a powerful moment for Danny—he realized he needed to make a change not only for himself, but to set a healthy example for his daughter.

SWAP VANITY FOR HEALTH.

It can be tempting to focus only on the physical transformation that takes place when you lose weight, but that's an easy way to lose sight of what's really important and to make yourself unhappy. Instead of setting goals like fitting into a particular clothing size or being the fittest person in your exercise class, focus on how eating nutritious foods and moving your body makes you feel strong and proud.

SWAP "GOOD/BAD" FOR "HEALTHY/ UNHEALTHY."

Using the words *good* and *bad* in relation to food and exercise conveys a sense of judgment that can easily make you feel like a good or bad *person*. We often reward ourselves when we've been "good" and punish ourselves when we've been "bad." These words only reinforce the all-or-nothing pattern that you're trying to escape.

SWAP SELF-LOATHING FOR SELF-ACCEPTANCE.

Accepting yourself, flaws and all, allows you to move forward to a place of caring and self-worth. Beating yourself up over past mistakes won't get you anywhere. The key to success is to focus on your future and to love yourself enough to commit to change.

Sometimes in order to help the people around you, you have to help yourself first. Season 8's Liz Young has a message for all the moms out there who put themselves at the bottom of their "to do" lists: "You are number one! Don't ever forget that. We grow up with our family as our first priority, but I'm no good to my family if I don't take care of myself first. I have to make time for myself." You may feel a little guilty or selfish about prioritizing your own needs at first, but eventually, just like healthy eating and exercise, making healthy lifestyle choices will simply become a part of your daily routine.

Getting Life Right

For Shay Sorrells of Season 8, losing weight and leading a healthy life will be about getting things right in her life. Her mother, who struggled with drug addiction, died 3 years ago at the age of 48.

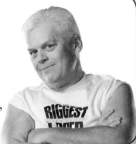

Jerry Skeabeck, Season 6

Getting healthy is like climbing a mountain. Once you get to the top, the view is inspiring!

Growing up, Shay spent time in foster homes and on the street with her mom. "She'll never see me have a child," says Shay. "She'll never see me break the cycle of addiction. She'll never see me break this mentality. She had a lot of struggles in her life, and some were passed to me. Some of them I overcame, but my struggle with food is the biggest one."

Shay is clear that her goals are long term, and she is committed to creating a life she can be proud

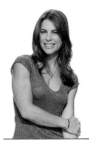

Trainer Tip: JILLIAN MICHAELS

Your health must come first. If it doesn't, your children will grow up thinking that anything they do for themselves is bad, because that's what they've learned from you. Do you want them to feel like that? Then show them something different.

of. "I want to inspire my family. So many people in my family are obese, are diabetic, and have high blood pressure. I want to see them live. I want to show them that a better life is possible."

Season 7 winner Helen Phillips says she is no longer hiding from life, staying at home because she has no clothes to wear to go out or because she's embarrassed about how she looks. Now she's looking in the mirror, she says, and beaming. "Now I'm just going to remember where I came from. What I accomplished. And do I really want to go back to being 257 pounds? Never."

"It's amazing how you can take something so broken and fix it," says Helen. "I know this is

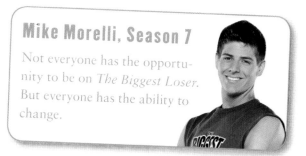

Mike Morelli, Season 7

Not everyone has the opportunity to be on *The Biggest Loser*. But everyone has the ability to change.

Jay Kruger, Season 5

Don't ever tell yourself you can't do something. You can do more than you think just by being positive.

something I will carry through my lifetime and pass along. Anyone who needs a hand, I'm willing to lend it. I'm going to be there, helping out girlfriends who have weight to lose."

So yes, the contestants on *The Biggest Loser* do have a shot at winning prizes, but more important, they also have a shot at a new, better life that they never imagined was possible. And so do you. Keep taking small steps and making Simple Swaps that enhance your health and the quality of your life. Create the life you want, and that you have every right to live.

It's a *Biggest Loser* World

From books to DVDs to meal plans to online support, *The Biggest Loser* brings life on the ranch into your own home with the same products and tools the contestants use to lose weight and maintain a healthy lifestyle. Go to www.biggestloser.com for more information.

Books

New York Times Bestsellers from Rodale Books

The Biggest Loser 30-Day Jump Start (2009)
The Biggest Loser Family Cookbook (2008)
The Biggest Loser Success Secrets (2008)
The Biggest Loser Fitness Program (2007)
The Biggest Loser Cookbook (2006)
The Biggest Loser Complete Calorie Counter (2006)
The Biggest Loser (2005)

DVDs

The Biggest Loser: Yoga (2008)
The Biggest Loser: Boot Camp (2008)
The Biggest Loser: Power Sculpt (2007)
The Biggest Loser: Cardio Max (2007)
The Biggest Loser: The Workout, Vol. 2 (2006)
The Biggest Loser: The Workout, Vol. 1 (2005)

Fitness Equipment

Body Bands
Fitness Mat
Resistance Bands
Stability Ball Kit: Stability Ball and Resistance Cord
Sculpt and Burn Kit: Weighted Water Ball and Jump Rope

Scales

The Biggest Loser Digital Weight Scales
The Biggest Loser Kitchen Scales
The Biggest Loser Nutritional Scales
The Biggest Loser Body Fat Scales

Appliances

The Biggest Loser Hand Blender and Chopping Jar
The Biggest Loser Chopper and Blender Prep System

The Biggest Loser Fruit and Vegetable Processor and Juicer

The Biggest Loser Blender and Smoothie Dispenser

The Biggest Loser Super Quick Multi Chopper and Storage System

The Biggest Loser Grill and Panini Press

The Biggest Loser Multi-Tier Food and Whole Grain Steamer

The Biggest Loser 10 Speed Blender

The Biggest Loser Food Chopper

The Biggest Loser Fruit and Vegetable Juice Extractor

The Biggest Loser Food Dehydrator

The Biggest Loser Icy Dessert Maker

The Biggest Loser Hand Blender with Whisk and Cup

The Biggest Loser Grill and Panini Maker

The Biggest Loser Steamer and Rice Cooker

The Biggest Loser Workout Drink Mixer

The Biggest Loser Protein

All Natural Chocolate Deluxe, 10-ounce can

All Natural Vanilla Bean, 10-ounce can

Red Raspberry, 10-ounce can, and Protein2Go (8 single-serving packets per box)

Blue Blueberry 10-ounce can and Protein2Go (8 single-serving packets per box)

The Biggest Loser 2010 Calendar

365 Day-to-Day Calendar with daily diet and exercise tips and success secrets to lose weight

The Biggest Loser Kitchen Stationery

Recipe organizers

Recipe cards

Kitchen stationery accessories

Online/Digital Kiosk

Biggest Loser Club from Rodale; www.biggestloserclub.com

Online subscription-based site based on the show includes lifestyle plan that creates customizable diet and fitness plans with access to community and experts.

The Biggest Loser Resort at Fitness Ridge

Now you can experience life at the ranch!

The Biggest Loser Meal Plan

www.biggestlosermealplan.com

Home delivery meal system designed by our doctors and experts

The Biggest Loser Workout Albums

The Biggest Loser Workout Mix: Top 40

The Biggest Loser Workout Mix: Top 40 Vol 2

The Biggest Loser Workout Mix: 80s Hits

The Biggest Loser Workout Mix: Country Hits

The Biggest Loser Workout Mix: Modern Rock Hits

The Biggest Loser Lifestyle Program for Nintendo Wii

The Biggest Loser Game

The Biggest Loser Wii Exercise Accessories

Contributors

CHERYL FORBERG, RD, is the nutritionist for *The Biggest Loser*. As cocreator of the eating plan, she has counseled each season's contestants on reaching their fitness and nutrition goals. A James Beard Award–winning chef, Cheryl brings a flavorful and fresh approach to eating for weight loss with a special emphasis on antiaging nutrition. She is the author of *Positively Ageless: A 28-Day Plan for a Younger, Slimmer, Sexier You* (Rodale, 2008). She also writes a weekly blog to share weight-loss tips and recipes at www.cherylforberg.com/blog. Cheryl is a graduate of the University of California, Berkeley. She lives in Napa, California.

MELISSA ROBERSON is the editor of BiggestLoserClub.com, the Web site that offers food, fitness, and exercise tips. She often visits the ranch and interviews trainers and contestants about their inspiring weight-loss journeys. She is a Web veteran, having worked on new media projects for Time Inc., the *New York Times*, News Corporation, Amazon.com, and BarnesandNoble.com. She lives in Hoboken, New Jersey.

Acknowledgments

To my coauthor and dear friend, Melissa Roberson: It is such a joy to work with you. I look forward to many more projects together.

I know we both thank everyone at NBC and Reveille—executives, producers, and crew of *The Biggest Loser*, especially Mark Koops and Chad Bennett—thank you for all the opportunities! I also want to thank Kat Elmore and Julie Ann Harris for making my visits and communiqués to the ranch so seamless.

To my peers on *The Biggest Loser* Medical Expert Team—Dr. Robert Huizenga, Dr. Michael Dansinger, Dr. Sean Hogan, and Sandy Krum—thanks so much for all your guidance and support.

Thanks to Dr. Barbara Sutherland of the University of California, Davis, and Marie Feldman, RD, for your nutritional wisdom and your friendship; to Geoff Jennings for your brilliant ideas and Web site support; to Lynn Arthur for your patience and creativity with recipe testing; and to my agent, Mary Lalli of Westport Entertainment, for your belief in my work and your support of my career.

Thanks to our trainers, Bob Harper and Jillian Michaels, who dedicate themselves tirelessly to the contestants and to the show.

Special thanks to our editor, Julie Will, at Rodale, for your clever ideas and mostly for always being there with just the right answers. I am proud to be working with you.

Biggest thanks to *The Biggest Loser* contestants—past and present, on-screen and off-screen. You all have such amazing stories; it has been a gift to know you and to work with each of you. Without you, this book wouldn't have been written. With you, a nation is inspired—thank you!

Cheryl Forberg RD

Index

Underscored page references indicate boxed text. **Boldface** references indicate photographs and illustrations.

Also available in the *New York Times* best-selling Biggest Loser series...

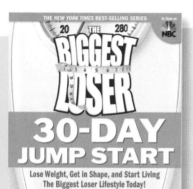

THE BIGGEST LOSER 30-DAY JUMP START
Lose Weight, Get in Shape, and Start Living The Biggest Loser Lifestyle Today!
The Biggest Loser Experts and Cast

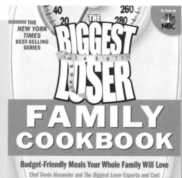

THE BIGGEST LOSER FAMILY COOKBOOK
Budget-Friendly Meals Your Whole Family Will Love
Chef Devin Alexander and The Biggest Loser Experts and Cast
with Melissa Roberson

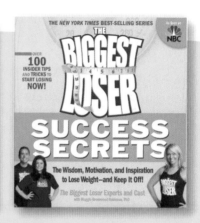

THE BIGGEST LOSER SUCCESS SECRETS
OVER 100 INSIDER TIPS AND TRICKS TO START LOSING NOW!
The Wisdom, Motivation, and Inspiration to Lose Weight—and Keep It Off!
The Biggest Loser Experts and Cast
with Maggie Greenwood-Robinson, PhD

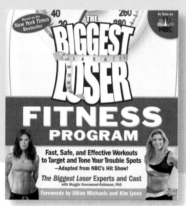

THE BIGGEST LOSER FITNESS PROGRAM
Fast, Safe, and Effective Workouts to Target and Tone Your Trouble Spots
—Adapted from NBC's Hit Show!
The Biggest Loser Experts and Cast
with Maggie Greenwood-Robinson, PhD
Forewords by Jillian Michaels and Kim Lyons

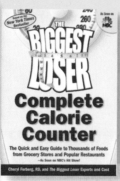

THE BIGGEST LOSER Complete Calorie Counter
The Quick and Easy Guide to Thousands of Foods from Grocery Stores and Popular Restaurants
—As Seen on NBC's Hit Show!
Cheryl Forberg, RD, and The Biggest Loser Experts and Cast

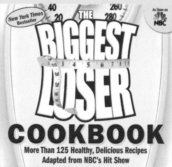

THE BIGGEST LOSER COOKBOOK
More Than 125 Healthy, Delicious Recipes Adapted from NBC's Hit Show
Chef Devin Alexander and The Biggest Loser Experts and Cast with Karen Kaplan
Foreword by Bob Harper and Kim Lyons

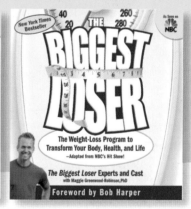

THE BIGGEST LOSER
The Weight-Loss Program to Transform Your Body, Health, and Life
—Adapted from NBC's Hit Show!
The Biggest Loser Experts and Cast
with Maggie Greenwood-Robinson, PhD
Foreword by Bob Harper

RODALE
LIVE YOUR WHOLE LIFE

Available wherever books are sold.

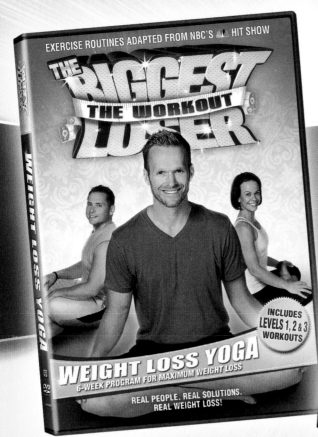
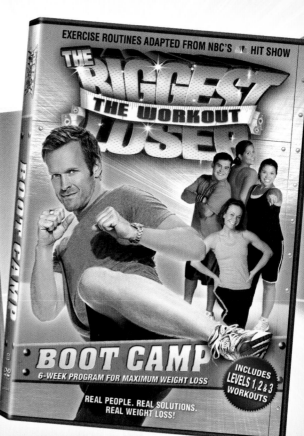

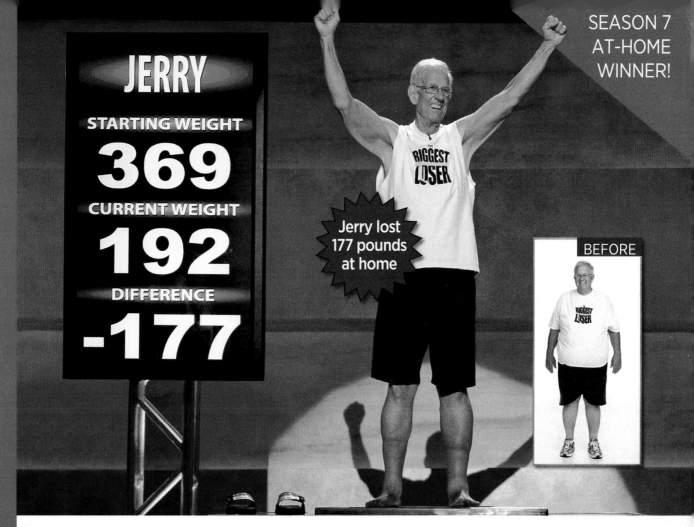

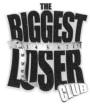

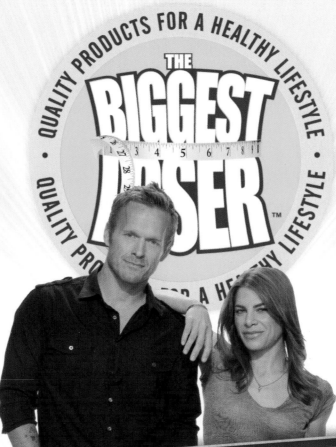

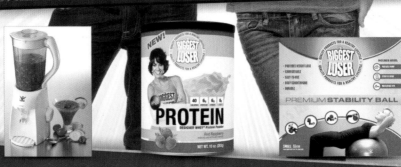

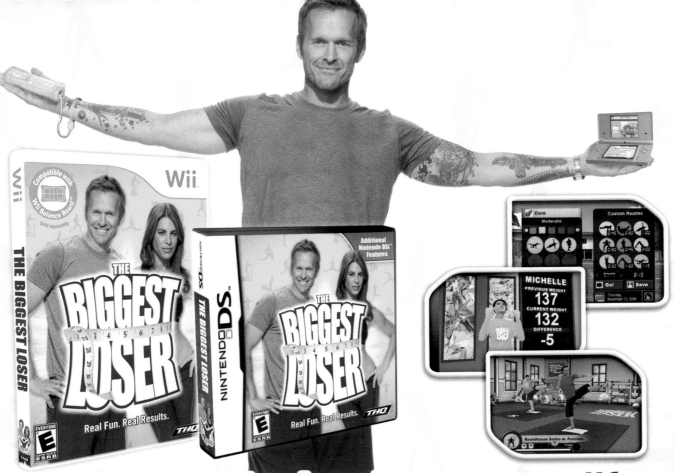

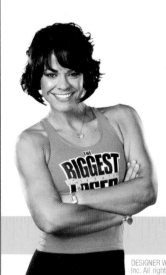
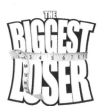

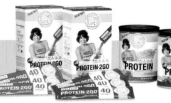
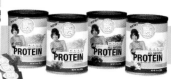
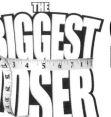
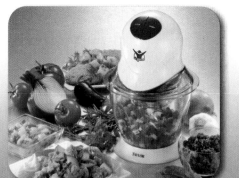